Conservative Management of Scoliosis Without Braces or Surgery

Published by
ROBERTS PUBLISHING COMPANY
606 E. Wisconsin Avenue
Oconomowoc, WI 53066

Author
R. B. MAWHINEY, D.C., D.I.S.R.C.

Copyright© Roberts Publishing Company (1998)

All rights reserved. No part of this book may be reproduced or transmitted in any form or by any means, electronic or mechanical, including photocopying, recording or by information storage and retrieval systems, without permission, in writing, from the publisher, except in a magazine or newspaper article referring to a specific part.

Printed in the United States of America
ISBN 0-931764-01-7

CONTENTS

Chapter One.................... 3
    Origin
    History
    Anatomy
    Classification

Chapter Two 13
    Screening
    Scoliometer
    Sam Machine
    Visual Examination
    Home Examination

Chapter Three 19
    X-ray Services
    Background
    History of Evaluation
    Reason for Measuring
    Hanging X-ray
    Lateral Bending Films

Chapter Four 29
    Bracing
    Types Available
    Rigid vs. Flexible

Chapter Five 47
    Treatment Procedures
    Medical vs. Conservative
    Cost Factors
    Expectations
    Length of Treatment

Chapter Six.................... 55
    Spinal Adjustments
    Restrictions
    Exercise
    Heel Supports/Orthotics
    Bilateral Weight Scales
    Weight Lifting

Chapter Seven 59
    Response by Age
    Infants
    Adolescents
    Young Adults
    Adults
    Seniors

Chapter Eight 63
    Published Research
    Reason for Publishing
    Articles

Chapter Nine 71
    Patient Questions
    1-800 Calls

Chapter Ten 83
    Board Certified Doctors
    Case Studies

Chapter Eleven 87
    Before and After X-rays

ACKNOWLEDGEMENTS

I am indebted to my patients and their families who have encouraged me to put into the printed word the thousands of questions I have answered over the years on the subject of scoliosis.

Several photos used in this book are used with permission of F. H. Barge, D.C., and Bradford Lonstein Ogilvie Winter, M.D. from their books on scoliosis.

AUTHORS COMMENTS

Since scoliosis is a conditions that does not require disability tags, a wheel chair or other outside signs of it's existence, it is thought by many to be an unimportant problem. In talking to the news media, the comment was always the same, when I would suggest a series on scoliosis, "it is not newsworthy". To the patient suffering with this condition, it involves their whole life. No one gives them the information they need to have to understand what is going on. This book is written in layman's language in an attempt to answer questions, give new hope and to dispel the demons of misinformation.

The same question has been uttered to me since I started obtaining results in 1952, and that is, "If it works why don't the medical doctors use the procedure?". I hope the reader will understand, after reading this book, that we are talking about an alternative treatment method and therefore, not available to the orthopedic surgeon. The treating doctor must be proficient in specific spinal segment adjusting. Only chiropractors receive that that type of training.

DEDICATED
TO
ALL THOSE WHO SUFFER IN SILENCE
AND DO NOT KNOW THAT
SOMETHING CAN BE DONE TO
RELIEVE THEIR SUFFERING.

Conservative Management

of

Scoliosis

Without Braces or Surgery

by

R. B. MAWHINEY, D.C., DIRECTOR

INTERNATIONAL SCOLIOSIS
RESEARCH CENTER, INC.

INTRODUCTION

Recently I had the chance to browse the internet and explore the web. One particular section, which caught my eye, was the Scoliosis Digest. The Scoliosis Digest is an area where individuals with scoliosis, or parents with children scheduled for surgery, can talk about their problems. It is basically a support group, for those who had surgery and want to know how to handle the pain and other problems that have developed. During the time I spent on the Web I was continually reminded of the number of patients still being scheduled for surgery. The most frequent comment heard was "How do I control the pain that is with me twenty-four hours a day?", "Where is there a doctor that will give me answers to my questions?" These, and many other questions were repeated daily by more people than I could count since this was only one Web site.

These questions should be directed to the doctor that performed the surgery, but in most instances the surgery was done years before and the doctor has since retired. The average patient does not realize the surgeon does their job and if it is successful they are finished and may not be available to answer questions later.

We, at the International Scoliosis Research Center, receive upwards of a hundred calls per month, from patients and their relatives, asking these same questions. Many of them are in a panic because of the stories they have heard and in some cases it is the information the doctor told them that has them frightened.

The knowledge that curvature of the spine exists goes back in history and the many ways of treating it included braces and even the rack. Unfortunately today some of the same treatment procedures are being used that were popular two hundred years ago.

The object of this book is to bring to the attention of the reader that conservative measures for the reduction of scoliosis has been available as a treatment protocol for almost seventy years. We will also provide answers to many questions concerning cause and effect. All the information put forth in this book is related to published works dealing with case studies and any case that is discussed as an individual case can be referenced by contacting the author.

> R. B. Mawhiney, D.C., D.I.S.C.
> Chairman of the Board
> International Scoliosis Research Center, Inc.

<u>Note:</u> Dr. Mawhiney has been in private practice, specializing in scoliosis treatment for over forty-five years and serves as a past, and present member, of the Continuing Education Postgraduate Faculty of ten colleges and has served as visiting professor at the Canadian Memorial Chiropractic College.

CHAPTER ONE

ETIOLOGY (cause)

The typical scoliosis is referred to as an "idiopathic scoliosis" by most of the members of the healing arts. The word "idiopathic" means unknown cause or unknown etiology. The majority of published articles and clinical studies deal with the idiopathic scoliosis. The problem with this concept is that the doctor writing the article or providing the treatment is admitting they are treating or discussing a condition that has an unknown cause and yet are providing information as to the treatment of this condition. How are you going to approach the proper treatment of a condition if you have no concept as to its cause? One of the problems that plague the use of braces and surgery is the continuous development of symptoms (residuals). The cause of the scoliosis is not approached by the use of braces and surgery.

Since we feel that God did not make any mistakes when He put the body together, the rule "that for every action there must be a reaction" will hold true. A doctor may say that a scoliosis is idiopathic and that is fine, since the doctor is saying they do not know the cause. That does not mean a cause does not exist. If the doctor states that they do not know the cause and will treat the symptoms or effects, then the patient is well informed. This is a prime rule in dealing with doctors. Always know what the doctor is doing or planning to do. I instruct patients to ask the doctor "why" every time they say something until they, as the patient, understand everything that is being done or will be done. You are hiring a person to do a job for you and you have the right to know everything possible. I point out to patients that they are expected to know more about scoliosis than the doctor. The doctor may have an idea how to treat it, but the patient should understand all the ramifications. I realize, probably more than the reader, the inability for the average doctor to fully discuss treatment effects and especially the orthopedic surgeon. I have found their general answer is, "you wouldn't understand".

The present treatment protocol (procedure) for the treatment of scoliosis by the medical profession, as presented by the Rochester Scoliosis Society is as follows:

>   10-20 degrees – wait and see
>   21-35 degrees – braces or casts
>   36 +   degrees – surgery

To break this down a few important points are necessary to explore.

1. *Why would anyone want to wait and see if a scoliosis gets worse?*

    Scoliosis of the spine is a progressive condition and only stops progressing based on the laws of physics. Based on this concept the doctor has no idea of how to treat it or stop it, so they might as well wait until it is bad enough so they can move to the next phase of treatment. Only one type of medical doctor deals with scoliosis and that is the orthopedic surgeon and, as his/her title suggests, surgery is their area of expertise.

2. *Who arbitrarily determined that braces would be used at this point in development?*

    The first generally accepted brace was developed by Dr. Blount, a Milwaukee, Wisconsin orthopedic surgeon. Braces had been used for over two hundred years, but his was developed in the early 1950's and made available to the medical profession. The concept used was that the spine was progressing and if the doctor put a brace on the outside of the body, somehow the body would decide that it had gone far enough and stop its progression. There are no two scoliosis exactly the same and as such no standard brace is going to consistently prevent progression. Dr. Blount stated clearly that "the brace will not correct the scoliosis but tends to prevent its progression." Every day thousands of patients are told by doctors, that "we will use the brace to see if we can reduce the curvature", which is a fallacy. We will discuss the cause of most scoliosis, but at this point it suffices to say that nothing is done to reduce the cause by the application of the brace, so it will continue to progress except in some minor Grade I curvatures.

3. *Surgery.*

It was then arbitrarily determined that when a curvature reaches 35 degrees it becomes dangerous, so "we" better operate. In the early 1950's and 1960's, it was determined that surgery would be applied after 45 degrees.

In the late fifties I was teaching a class of doctors, for board certification, in Long Island, New York. When I discussed the medical policy of surgery at 45 degrees I was corrected by a doctor who had a brother working on the staff of one of the teaching hospitals. He told me that his brother had told him that the 45 degree requirement for scoliosis surgery had been reduced to 35 degrees because "they had too many residents that had not had experience in that type of surgery and this provided more patients." I could question that logic except when I graduated in 1953, normal blood pressure was 100 over your age. Then when a new diuretic was developed it was changed to 140/80. In a medical publication in the 1980's, a move was made to lower the "normal" blood pressure to 135/85. That would also sell a lot of diuretics. My point is that the original reason for suggesting surgery had to do with the concept that a curvature over 35 degrees could eventually cause compression on the heart and lungs which could cause cardiopulmonary collapse. Recent published articles have indicated you would have to have up to 110 degrees of curvature before you would effect cardiopulmonary collapse. Do you think this latest published information has reduced the number of surgeries? Guess again.

The formation of the hump is also used as a reason for the intervention of surgery, but there are other ways to deal with that problem if the scoliosis is noted early enough. The average person does not understand that the medical and chiropractic colleges do not provide procedures for treating scoliosis. The doctor learns about scoliosis and then learns something about treatment in their clinical training, but usually feel it will be taken care of by specialists. Consequently, the family doctor, pediatrician, etc. have no idea how to treat these cases and unfortunately have a lot of incorrect information they mistakenly pass on to their patients.

Somewhere along the line people were led to believe all doctors knew everything about all conditions and since we deal with a lot of ego's, many doctors do not want to dispel that myth. In all my years in practice I always hear about "their" doctor being the best in the area. If you stop and think about it they can't all graduate in the top of the class. This is why I am happy to see people who are asking questions of the doctor and doing their research into scoliosis so they can determine the correct approach to treatment. If your pediatrician, family doctor, or family chiropractor suggests treatment for scoliosis, always ask what training they received in scoliosis. For chiropractors, they should not treat the case unless they have had postgraduate work in the subject. Many doctors become upset if you ask for proof, but if they have had the training they should be happy to show you what advanced training they received. You are trusting your body and your health to this person and have a right to know. Always check credentials.

The International Scoliosis Research Center has, through sixty years of research and case studies, determined the cause of scoliosis as follows:

85% of all scoliosis are caused by trauma (blow-fall) to the pelvic mechanism (buttocks) in the formative years from 5 to 10 years of age with postural adaptation determining the extent of progression. When God designed the body it was determined the head must be balanced over the tailbone in order to maintain balance (homeostasis). The sacrum, or tail bone is the foundation upon which the spine rests. Weight is transferred from the body into the tailbone and then into the legs and down to the feet. The spine provides contour to the body but primarily protects the spinal cord from damage. Each vertebra, there are twenty-four of them from the base of the skull to the tailbone, can move in seven directions but primarily rotate to allow us to turn our bodies in different directions while still keeping our feet flat on the ground. When the pelvis is traumatized we usually have a displacement of the sacrum (tailbone) on one side. This causes the foundation upon which the spine rests to become lower on one side. Due to the laws of biomechanics, the body of the lowest freely movable vertebra will always rotate to the low side of its foundation.

In the treatment of scoliosis it is imperative to determine if there is a short leg on one side since all the treatment in the world directed to the spine will not correct a short leg. By placing a brace on the spine the actual cause, which may be a short leg, is being ignored. Once the cause is determined, it is easy to set up a treatment schedule to fit the situation.

In the area of physics we find the body will attempt to keep the head balanced over the tailbone in order to maintain proper posture. If the pelvis is lower on one side, the vertebra in the lower back, began to rotate to the low side. Due to the design of the lower vertebra (lumbar), the front of the vertebra is thicker than the rear part. This has to do with the contour of the spine but also has a direct effect on the curve formation of the spine. As the vertebra rotate towards the low side they actually build up a high point which causes the next higher vertebra to rotate the opposite direction. This way we can look at an early developing scoliosis and tell where the next curve will start.

When the body is in the normal, or anatomical position, the head is over the sacrum and the body weight is evenly distributed to both legs. When there is a pelvic imbalance, such as a short leg, it forces the high weight distribution to one side further increasing the developing of the scoliosis. This is why a scoliosis is a progressive condition and waiting to see what will happen will only allow it to get worse.

Many times you will hear a doctor say it is a "congenital" scoliosis, which implies the person was born with the condition or inherited it from their parents. The definition of scoliosis requires a lateral deviation of the spine with elements of vertebral rotation. It is a rare situation that would cause this effect because at birth the vertebra are small osseous centers held together with ligaments. It is not until the child puts weight on the spine that the vertebra will start to rotate to one side. If a child is born with boney deformities then this will predispose to the development of the scoliosis when the child begins to walk. The etiology in that case would be osseous deformity, not congenital. If a child suffers an injury to any part of the lower extremity an uneven foundation develops and we have the start of a scoliosis. It is imperative for any child that suffers a trauma to the lower extremity be checked by someone who understands the biomechanics of scoliosis progression to be sure nothing develops from the injury. A medical doctor does not have the understanding to determine the effects of a trauma of that nature. The medical doctor is trained to treat disease and since scoliosis is not a disease, it is outside their field.

Many times the doctor will say that the scoliosis is only minor and of no consequence. Scoliosis is a progressive condition and will only get worse unless the cause is corrected. It would be the same as telling a woman "its only a little pregnancy, don't worry about it." Do not accept the opinion of a doctor unless they have specialty training in scoliosis. An internist, pediatrician or family doctor may recognize a scoliosis but do not have the training to treat it or give opinions. The orthopedic surgeon is the one who has patients referred to them for most scoliosis cases. Remember, they are surgeons and that is the area in which they work. They are trained to treat scoliosis with braces and surgery and do not have any other procedure available to them.

We have classified scoliosis into two distinct categories; functional and structural. Both of them have a lateral deviation from the midline with elements of vertebral rotation. The structural scoliosis has osseous deformities which the functional does not. We further class them into seven simple classes, each with a prescribed treatment plan. The treatment plans have been in effect since the early 1930's and have been modified with new technology as it develops.

SCOLIOSIS POSTER

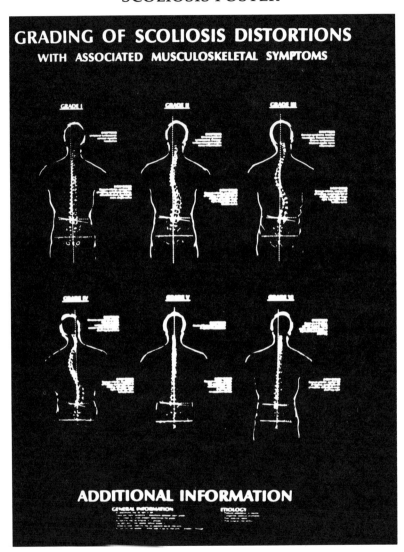

Poster showing the progression of scoliosis from first pelvic change to grade IV.

A doctor should be able to satisfy your questions as to why you, or your child, have the scoliosis and what you can expect in the future. Is it a fast moving scoliosis or do you have time to get it under control with restrictions or exercises? If the doctor can not answer the questions you have you should go to someone else. Just because the doctor may have a good reputation does not always make them the best for you. You have to feel comfortable and do not let the doctor talk down to you. This is particularly true of one type of doctor who implies that the patient is not smart enough to know what they are talking about. If the doctor explains to you there are things that are not understood about scoliosis it may mean they do not understand it since scoliosis has been well understood since the late thirties. Trust your judgement and if the doctor suggests surgery "ALWAYS" get another opinion, but not from a medical doctor since that is the only direction they can suggest you follow.

There never has been any justification for the *'wait and see'* procedure. We have reached an age where people are better educated and demand better understanding of any condition that they may be diagnosed as having. The doctor may have good intentions, but if the only thing you have been taught to use is surgery that is what you will suggest.

The prime purpose of this book is to inform the average patient of the functions of the body, with scoliosis, and to allow them to use good judgment in determining the direction of the treatment they are about to receive. You should expect results in 90 days, or a good explanation that you can accept if the results are not as planned. If you understand the cause and the direction that the scoliosis is going, it will be easier to discuss the case with the doctor.

CHAPTER TWO

SCREENING

In the late seventies the United States government decided that all grade school children must be evaluated for the presence of scoliosis. The screening was to be done by doctors so that early detection might prevent the development of an advanced scoliosis. The medical profession is divided into specialities, so it was felt that the best doctors for the job would be the orthopedic surgeons. The protocol for treatment of scoliosis by the orthopods has always been to 'wait and see', then braces and then surgery.

The first few years found a lot of screenings being run but more and more of them were being conducted by the school nurse since the orthopods did not have the time to devote to this program. Later, in the 1980's I was told a directive went to the state school superintendent to discontinue the screening since not enough cases were found to warrant care. In other words, there were not enough cases to warrant bracing or surgery since there was nothing they could to do prevent an early case from getting worse. By transferring the screening over to school nurses the quality of screening suffered since scoliosis screening was never a part of their training. The nurses, though dedicated, had little understanding about the cause and progression of scoliosis. It is a condition that does not evoke a great amount of sympathy since there is little outward signs until it becomes quite severe.

People associated with the condition in their family find it difficult to receive answers since the condition is not considered to be a "visible" problem, and therefore TV and radio stations have little interest in doing any investigating reports.

One hears a variety of reports as to the frequency of scoliosis in the population. I received a flyer this morning from a local hospital and find they are using the same "10% of the population" they were using forty-five years ago when I graduated. Medically, this does not mean anything since their definition of a scoliosis may be considered as any curve of ten degrees or more. Since God designed the body to be in proper alignment a ten degree deviation would become extensive. I consider any deviation, from the midline, whether it be 3 degrees or more, is a scoliosis. The measurement of 1-2 degrees is considered to be a measurable error.

We at the International Scoliosis Research Center find that 99% of our patients have a scoliosis and for the last forty-five years, I would say that over 90% of the patients that enter a chiropractors office show some sign of a scoliosis. I have seen hundreds of cases with curvatures measuring over thirty degrees denied treatment because they were not ready for surgery. The average patient does not realize that doctors, (chiropractors-medical-osteopathic) graduate from school prepared to take the national and state exams. They learn about diseases and treatments in their internship and residency. Based on this point few doctors know anything at all about scoliosis. You should only listen to a doctor that can prove they have had specialty training in the field of scoliosis. It is hard to imagine, but a large majority of doctors, in all disciplines, may say "let this condition get worse than we might be able to do something with it". The screening programs have been reinstated the last few years and are now being done more by chiropractors. This is only acceptable if the chiropractor has had special training. If this is being done in your school have the administration check the doctors credentials. The <u>parent</u> is still the best person for screening the child.

Screening procedures for parents:
If you are dealing with a child under four years of age have them stand, facing away from you, dressed in underpants. If you can see two indentations at the small of the back, these are known as sacral dimples. These will normally leave after the child reaches six years

of age. If one of the dimples is deeper than the other you already have a scoliosis starting.

If the child is in grade school, have them face the same way dressed in their underwear and notice if one arch (in the foot) is flatter than the other. This will normally indicate a fallen arch and will cause one leg to be shorter than the other one and this will predispose to a scoliosis.

If it is a teenage girl, check them in a bra and underwear facing away from you. The most noticeable sign is the bra strap will not be level. You will also notice the panties will be lower on one side. The shoulder will be higher on the same side and the head may be tilted. This is not always seen in the school screening since the ones doing the screening are not trained to look for the right signs. If you have not checked earlier, also check the arches in the feet. Boys can be checked the same way but their hips and shoulders will be the best indication.

Do not let the family doctor be the only one to examine for a scoliosis since they are not trained for this type of condition.

The doctors academic standing in class study does not determine the quality of the doctor. I feel patient relationship and a desire to help are the best qualities.

Sometimes parents ask about a child having their feet toe in or out. I do not treat this type of case until they reach age three since it takes that much time for the pelvic areas to stabilize and then we can determine if the problem is in the feet or in the pelvis. If a child is born with any type of lower extremity deformity, such as a club foot or dislocated hip, then a scoliosis will most likely occur.

We recognize that teens have a postural problem and most parents have given up long ago on getting them to stand straight. I have found they respond to seeing a severe scoliosis, so if you take them to your chiropractor, they may be able to understand what poor posture can lead to.

When a child is facing away from you, look at the head to see if it tilts to one side. Is one shoulder lower than the other? Does the forearm on one side touch the hip while the other hangs free? These are all physical signs that any parent can recognize and is a far more complete scoliosis exam than you could get at any school. Have you had to alter skirts or slacks for variations in length? That is another good sign a scoliosis has started. Have the child face away from you and have them turn their head as far as they can, first in one direction and then in the other. If they can turn more in one direction than the other it may indicate that the lower spine has already started to rotate in the same direction.

If they have been diagnosed as having a scoliosis, or you have been unfortunate to have a medical doctor tell you to watch it develop, you may try another procedure. With a washable pencil, mark the boney segment of the spine. Then have them hang by their hands, while facing away from you, and see if the spine straightens.

Some chiropractors use a machine known as the SAM machine which can give you an indication if a scoliosis is present. You can also use two scales. Have them stand on two scales, looking straight ahead and see of the weight remains balanced with about the same amount on each foot. This is not a simple test. We use a computerized scale in our office to determine weight distribution.

There is an instrument known as a Scoliometer that some doctors have that can also help you determine if there is a curvature. It measures the height of the shoulder, hips and head tilt in degrees or millimeters.

Check the heel on their shoes, to see if they are warn unevenly. If you see that they are uneven you should then check the postural areas I mentioned earlier in this chapter because it is apparent the child is not carrying their weight evenly and a curve may be developing. In one of my published articles "Is Scoliosis Screening In Our Schools Missing The Mark?" (1), I reported on school screenings in three Wisconsin communities, involving over three thousand children, that had shown less than three percent with a scoliosis that the nurse could identify. The general opinion, of those who work with scoliosis, indicate that at least ten percent of the population has this condition, and I say that close to fifty percent of grade school children show some lateral deviation of the spine. As I said before, medically they have to see at least ten degrees of change before they can class it as a scoliosis, and to me any lateral movement must be stopped. God created it straight so that is where it should be.

After evaluating thousands of children and adults for scoliosis during the last forty-five years, I still feel the parent is the best person to do the screening. Why should you have to ask a doctor, who knows less about the subject than you do, to do something that you are far more qualified to do? If you have read this book to this point, you already know more than the average doctor about this condition, now you want to find a doctor to treat the condition. Remember, you are hiring someone to perform a service, so ask the right questions.

CHAPTER THREE

X-RAY SERVICES

This chapter deals with x-ray services. Since x-rays were discovered in 1895 they have continued to be fine tuned for specific procedures and evaluations. An x-ray is a two plane view of an object in various shades of white to black. A doctor's ability to understand what the x-ray is telling them is directly related to their experience and training. The average medical doctor, based on information from the Wisconsin Medical College, has only a thirty hour non-required course in x-ray in their senior year. One of the reasons for this is the formation of the specialist in radiology who can read the x-ray for the doctor. On the other hand a chiropractor, in the state of Wisconsin, is required to have three hundred hours of x-ray training before they can take the state board. I bring this point up to let the reader know that the family medical doctor is not trained in scoliosis and the reading of x-rays dealing with scoliosis. Just because the chiropractor has all that training does not qualify them to treat scoliosis, but it does qualify them to recognize it and to give an opinion.

More often we find the medical doctor ordering a CAT scan or a MRI for evaluation of a scoliosis. Generally a CAT scan is used to determine the presence of tissue pathology. In forty-five years of treating over four thousand scoliosis cases I have never seen a case with either bone or soft tissue pathology in a scoliosis. That does not mean it does not exist, but it does tell you that you should have plenty of evidence for the need to spend that kind of money on a test that is of little value in a scoliosis case. Scoliosis is a musculoskeletal condition, not a disease, therefore a standard x-ray will give any qualified doctor all the information they require to determine a treatment program. The average doctor is not aware of the etiology (cause) of scoliosis so they order many tests to rule out other factors. I do not feel it is necessary to subject a child to all these tests. You may not feel the expense is a problem, because the insurance company pays the bill. Remember, any expense charged to the insurance company is made up in the premium.

A proper x-ray of a scoliosis case involves the taking of two films, a full spine front to back view, that includes the full pelvis, and a full spine lateral view that includes the pelvis. If there are two or more curves, a hanging x-ray is required. (2), (3) Full spine films were first introduced into the study of scoliosis in the 1930's at Logan College of Chiropractic in St. Louis, Missouri. Logan College was founded on the principle that a scoliosis could be reduced with conservative management. It was necessary to take full spine films because information available in the pelvis was needed to determine the treatment procedures. At that time most films were what we call "sectionals" and they just viewed a smaller part of the body.

One of the questions that they became aware of in the 1930's was that there had to be a way for the doctor to know if the curvature could be reduced before the treatment began. Since the curvature, in eighty-five percent of the cases, is caused by a pelvic unleveling they had to devise a method by which the pelvis could return towards a normal position. They devised a "hanging" x-ray (3) to evaluate the changes that might take place. When God designed the body, the head had to be balanced over the sacrum or tailbone. As I said earlier, the vertebra will rotate to the low side of their foundation and the curves will develop. When we hang by our hands the weight is taken off the spine and the vertebra tend to rotate back toward the mid-line. As they rotate back to the mid-line the curves reduce accordingly. By measuring the curves in the gravity (standing) position and then measuring the curves in the hanging film we can determine how much reduction is possible under conservative management. The "hanging" procedure requires the patient to hang by their hands for an accumulated time of two minutes and the x-ray is taken while they are hanging.

I have had patients who have seen the results of the hanging film, and then realize how much their curve could be reduced, ask "why the medical doctors didn't take the same kind of film so they too could see if the curve could be reduced." First, you remember the medical profession classes their scoliosis as idiopathic. Second, the prescribed procedure calls for the doctors to take lateral bending films because that procedure is in the acceptable protocol. Doctors do not change the "accepted procedure" unless it has been clinically tested and then accepted by the profession. It is interesting to note that many chiropractic colleges take lateral bending films, instead of hanging films, because they wish to follow the medical procedures.

Medically, since the turn of the century, the medical profession has labeled the majority of scoliosis cases as idiopathic. One of the reasons is that they do not consider the pelvis, which is the foundation upon which the spins rests, as an integral part of the scoliosis syndrome. If your house is starting to lean in one direction you would immediately check to see if the foundation is sinking. When you consider that the spine rests on the sacrum and as the sacrum becomes lower on one side, the spine will rotate to the low side of its foundation. If you do not x-ray the pelvis (foundation) how do you get the spine to rotate back to the mid-line? Scoliosis progression is predictable and when a full spine film is taken, it can be determined how fast the curve is moving and what chance there is to reduce the curves.

Rescheduled x-rays, those taken after a period of care, are usually taken with orthotics or heel lifts in the shoe, so the actual effect of the supports may be measured. In recent years we have produced a study showing the predictability of scoliosis reduction by the extent of reduction in the hanging film. The hanging film is a standard procedure for all chiropractors board certified in scoliosis care.

The importance of the hanging x-ray has been demonstrated since 1939, but as of now is only taught through the postgraduate educational department of the colleges. If a doctor does not take a postgraduate class in scoliosis they are never exposed to this procedure. I have attempted to have the spinal center, located in Minneapolis, Minnesota investigate the results of this procedure, but to no avail. I hope the reader will understand how important it is to take a hanging film so when you see your doctor, insist on having this taken to determine if the spine can be reduced without bracing or surgery. If the surgeon wants to perform surgery, ask for the hanging film. If they do not understand or do not have the facility available, call us and we will try to find someone for you. Scoliosis is not fatal so do not be rushed into surgery without the proper x-rays.

When we take a film we measure each vertebra to determine the amount of rotation, the speed of rotation and the direction. If you have films from your medical doctor, ask to see the amount of rotation. Ask the doctor to tell you how fast it is moving and to tell you how long it has been since it started. If the doctor can not answer these questions, how are they going to know how to treat it?

The hanging film then tells us which vertebra are freely movable and what area will change first. This is important if the doctor is to apply the right procedure to get the best results. We look for an ideal reduction of 50%, in the hanging film, but any reduction in the hanging film is a positive. If the hanging film does not show any reduction, then you know before you start that any change will be accepted.

A point that has bothered me as a chiropractor is how the doctors and hospitals will take x-rays without proper gonadal protection. This means protecting the breast and genitals from radiation. There are adapters in use today that will allow any x-ray machine to have the proper protection. You parents, do not let them take x-rays without protection for your children. If they say "we do not use any protectors" then you say "no x-ray". I have not seen an x-ray from any of the hospitals in the metropolitan area of Milwaukee, Wisconsin that have any protection and it is up to the parents to see that this procedure is implemented to protect the future of our children. If the doctor indicates that protection is not necessary, say good-bye, and walk away.

Have the x-rays explained to you so that you understand the problem at hand. If the doctor uses words you do not understand, ask them to explain it until you do understand. I can not say it often enough, you are paying someone to perform a service for you and you have a right to understand what is going on. I have always made it a policy to ask the parents what area of expertise they may have so I might use the explanation in a familiar area of understanding. When I talk to an engineer I use construction of a building as an example. If it is a mother, who is at home there are all types of examples one can use and analogies that will fit the explanation.

A doctor is like the captain of a ship and does not like to be told what to do, but you have a right to have it explained so you may understand the problem.

Various treatment procedures require different x-ray views. We find, after seventy years of working with scoliosis cases, that three views, full spine, lateral and hanging are the maximum necessary. In some cases there may be some areas of pathology that require a spot film. These should be explained to you so you may be aware of a possible problem. We follow up with a full spine AP and hanging films in 90-120 days and if the reduction of the curves are adequate we may not x-ray for six months. It makes no sense to x-ray every three months just to see if it is getting worse. We evaluate to see what changes will have to be made in the treatment procedures. This first three month period is to stop the progression and to start the reduction process. If there is no reduction then a change in procedure is necessary. It is not possible to reduce all cases, but unless you try, instead of just waiting and watching, nothing is being accomplished.

If a doctor wants to wait six months before x-raying and is not applying any treatment, I would suspect their motives. Any case under a treatment schedule should show some signs of change in a three month period. If the doctor states that they do not want to expose you to any more radiation then they are not protecting you enough in the first place.

HANGING X-RAY

A hanging x-ray allows the doctor to determine how much reduction is possible without braces or surgery, using conservative measures.

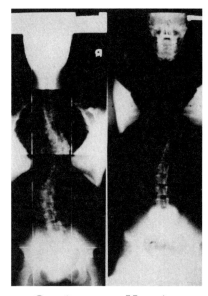

Gravity Film   Hanging Film

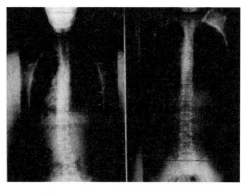

Gravity Film   Hanging Film

24

HANGING X-RAY

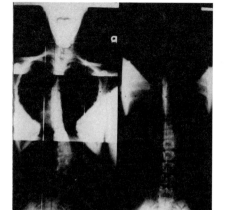

Gravity Film   Hanging Film

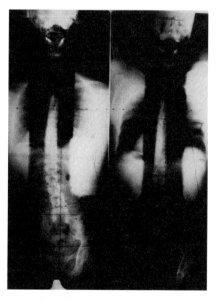

Gravity Film   Hanging Film

Hanging x-ray showing a reduction from 27 degrees to 16 degrees with a reduction in pelvic unleveling.

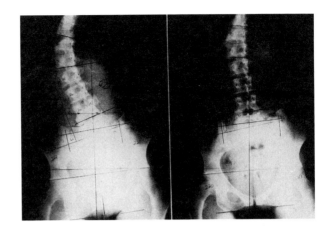

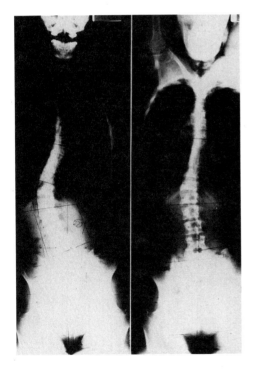

Hanging x-ray of a Grade IV left lumbar rotatory scoliosis. Reduction in hanging film over 30%.

STANDING A.P. LUMBAR X-RAY

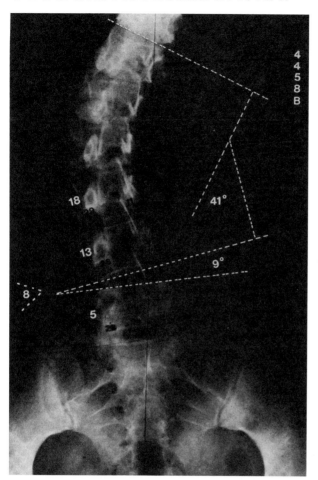

This A.P. standing x-ray presents a left rotatory lumber scoliosis initiated by a left sacral inferiority. Then due to balance factors or trauma a disc block subluxation occurred between L4 and L5. Notice that L4 is rotated (body left) 8mm away from the open side of the disc wedge in relation to L5. The angle of the disc wedge is 9 degrees and the Cobb angle is 41 degrees.

HANGING A.P. LUMBAR X-RAY

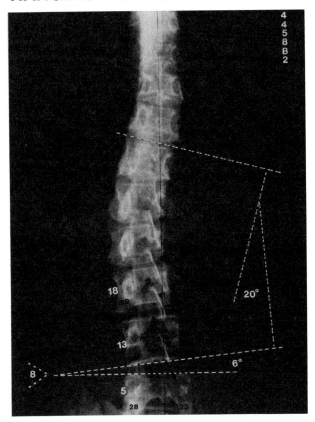

This is a hanging x-ray of the person on the previous page. Notice the remarkable 21 degree change in the Cobb angle and yet only a 3 degree change in the disc wedge between L4 and L5. If the disc block disc wedge had remained the same 9 degrees (black lines and angle) the Cobb angle would have been approximately 24 degrees. So actually the Cobb angle change has been accomplished by the change in the disc wedges between all of the lumbar vertebrae. The identity of the disc block subluxation has not been altered, the disc block subluxation's rotational disrelationship and wedge remains unchanged.

CHAPTER FOUR

BRACING

Records from the seventeenth and eighteenth centuries indicate various types of braces have been applied to people with spinal curvatures on a continuing basis. There are even pictures of patients being placed on the "rack" and being stretched to reduce the curve. The thought was if they could push it back in the middle it should stay there. (Fig. 1)

There have been problems with this system since its inception. When Dr. Blount of Milwaukee, Wisconsin came out with the first readily accepted body brace in the 1950's, it was felt to be the answer. Even those who developed the first braces did not seem to understand the laws of physics. If you do not address the cause, how are you going to apply treatment? One analogy is like trying to stop the dog from wagging its tail by holding on to the tail. They forget it is the dog that is causing the tail to wag and on a similar vein it is the unleveled pelvis that is causing the spine to curve and the placing of a brace on the spine, which is the result of the unleveling, would be the same as holding onto the tail of the dog.

Dr. Blount stated that the brace was meant to prevent progression of the curve. This would be fine if the curve presence was due to a spinal problem and not a pelvic one. Since eighty-five percent are due to pelvic problems the brace becomes unnecessary. The brace can cause other problems:

1. Compression of abdominal viscera is caused by squeezing the abdominal area while trying to reduce the curve.
2. Increased pressure on the stomach area which interferes with digestion and may cause heartburn.
3. Decrease in kidney function.
4. Increase in sodium retention, which is related to the kidneys.

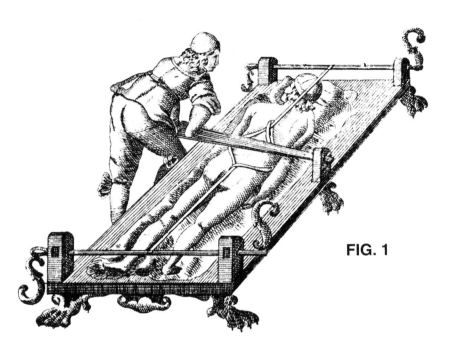

FIG. 1

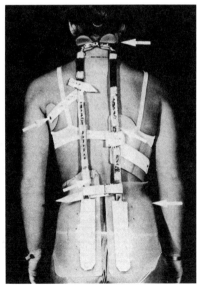

FIG. 2 — Posterior view of a CTLSO demonstrates the transverse forces that can be generated (from cephalad to caudad) with the neck ring, axillary sling, thoracic pad, lumbar pad, and the pelvic mold.

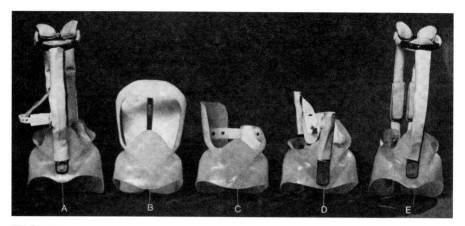

FIG. 3 – Five basic patterns of spinal orthosis can be modified as required. (a), CTLSO (Milwaukee brace) with left lumbar pad and right thoracic pad used for s-shaped scoliosis, (b), TLSO used in thoracic and thoracolumbar curves, (c), Modified TLSO with left lumbar pad for lumbar curves, (d), The extension on this modified TLSO provides a more open design and counteracts the left lumbar pad's tendency to right trunk tilt., (e), CTLSO for thoracic kyphosis.

5. Decrease in total lung volume, which can effect the overall systemic function of the body.
6. Treatment with body braces can cause psychological disturbances that can manifest themselves into adult life creating various neuroses.

(Note:) We have had children come to the office totally dependent upon the brace to the extent they were afraid that the spine would collapse if they removed the brace for any period of time. Some doctors impart this fear to the patient and actually create this phobia.

As stated before, the standard medical procedure calls for a "wait and see" period until the curve reaches twenty-three degrees. Bracing is to prevent it from increasing to thirty-five degrees. Then surgery after it reaches thirty-five degrees. It is interesting to note we have many patients come to our office after they have been scheduled for surgery to see if we can help them. They may have a curvature over fifty degrees and still the orthopod has scheduled them to wear a brace for up to six months. Why, if surgery is the only approach the doctor feels can be done, would you place a child in a brace for three to six months?

The study of biomechanics indicate the vertebra will always rotate to the low side of their foundation, so why brace the spine and not do anything to the pelvis. Pictures of the various braces in use today give you an idea of how they are used on children. It is interesting to read on the WEB the problems people have with the braces and the help they are seeking from others in the same boat. I always wondered why a person would go on the internet to ask these questions instead of asking their doctor? I asked some orthopedic surgeons and they said, "I do not have time to answer questions like that and I refer them to a therapist or nurse." In other words, they do not know what to do to stop the skin rash, abrasions and irritation caused by the brace.

When a brace is applied the main pressure is brought against the thoracic spine (rib cage area). In most cases this is the secondary curve and not the primary curve that is causing the trouble. There are two pads placed on the hip bones, for stability, and an adjustable pad placed on the upper lateral curve. The vertebra rotate, which helps the curve to move laterally. Applying a pad on the external surface to move it medial (towards the center), does not reduce the rotation of the vertebra and therefore, is subject to failure before it starts. No one wants these curves to increase and people accept the brace as a means without understanding the loss of time and the expense involved.

The average doctor will monitor the thoracic curve, which will usually move faster, particularly in the female, and place a pad at that point. There are many types of braces available to the doctor and as you can see by the pictures they are applied to all ages. Many doctors will suggest the brace with the "halo" attachment which is totally contrary to the laws of physics. The cervical spine is the last area to rotate in the average scoliosis and by making the cervical rigid you create more problems than you can imagine. First of all, God created the spine to be flexible and to hold it in a rigid position will cause the development of boney changes in the small joint areas of the cervical spine. It will cause the development of headaches, neck strain, and sleeping problems along with personality changes. If you do not believe this try walking around for six months in a simple neck brace and see how your personality changes. In this case, we are talking about children.

Most of the books on the market today deal with bracing and surgery. Two books, "Stopping Scoliosis" by Nancy Schommer, a science writer, deals with bracing and surgery. "The Scoliosis Handbook" by M. Neuwirth, M.D. is far more specific in the description of the pre- and post-surgical situations. Neither book offers any alternative to the treatment of scoliosis by specific spinal adjustment, even though that procedure has been an integral part of the scoliosis scene for over seventy years. A third book, "Moe's Textbook of Scoliosis and Other Spine Deformities" by Bradford, Lonstein, Ogilvie and Winter, is used extensively by orthopedic surgeons as a guide. It does not consider any treatment other than bracing and surgery.

COMPLICATIONS

Orthotic treatment is not without potential complications and problems. Although usually mild and transient from a physical standpoint, both somatic and psychological changes can occur when orthotic treatment is elected. Compression of abdominal viscera is an invariable companion of a properly fitting TLSO.

Increased intragastric pressure may result in reflux esophagitis. A decrease in glomerular filtration rate and effective renal blood flow has also been noted. Although reversible with removal of the brace, this tendency toward sodium retention could be measured in certain patients even after four to twelve months of brace treatment. A slight decrease in total lung volume has been noted in patients wearing the CTLSO; however, there has been no significant effect on the vital capacity. The circumferential fitting TLSO has more restriction of thoracic expansion than does the CTLSO, and prolonged wearing can produce a "tubular thorax" deformity.

Brace treatment in the adolescent can produce psychological disturbances that are measurable into adult life. Self-image in adolescents is difficult to evaluate, but it is an important factor in compliance with brace wearing, and it also affects whether the patient is satisfied with the cosmetic result following years of brace treatment. Orthosis patients in general have a less favorable outlook towards their body image than do surgery patients.

CASTING

This is a more radical procedure than the bracing since the full body case is normally worn for up to six months and the residuals to the procedure are quite extensive. In this case the patient may not remove the cast, under any circumstances. It has been said that when Dr. Blount was asked why he wanted his patients to wear the Milwaukee brace for twenty-three hours he said, "because they will not wear it for twenty-four hours". With the casting system they are forced to wear it for six months without removing it. Casting has the same success rate as the body brace, which is a negative number. The basic principles of physics are the same for bracing or casting, and casting is the worse of the two. The object of this book is not to tell you when to use braces or surgery, but to inform you of the aspects of scoliosis and to realize there are other ways to treat scoliosis without braces or surgery.

TRACTION

Over thirty years ago a procedure was introduced where in the patient would have pins placed in their skull and both knees. They would then be placed in traction to stretch the spine. Remember my mentioning the "rack" earlier, well this does sound a little like the rack, but only a twentieth century version. When I mentioned this to a faculty member at the Medical School of Wisconsin, and told him of the many problems this will cause without correcting the spinal problem, he answered, "this is not as bad as the procedure where they use up to 120 pounds of cervical traction to try and straighten the spine. They actually tear the meninges" (covering of the spinal cord).

FULL BODY CAST

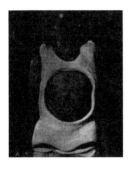
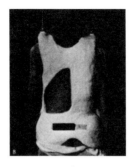
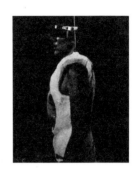

FULL BODY CASE
WITH OCCIPITOL SUPPORT

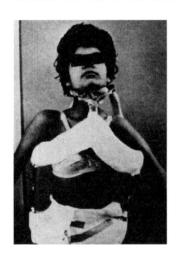

PREPERATION FOR
FULL BODY CAST

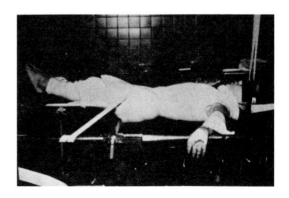

"HALO" ATTACHMENT TO THE SKULL

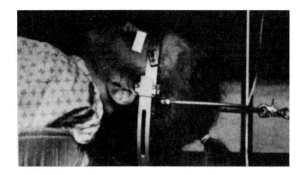

PELVIC CAST WITH "HALO" ATTACHMENT

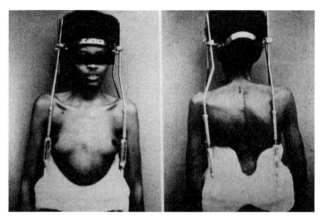

SUPPORT BRACE FOR AN INFANT

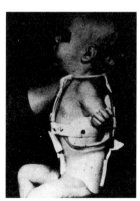

CASTING WITH A "HALO" AND SURGERY

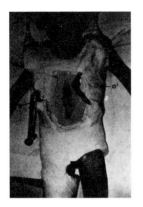 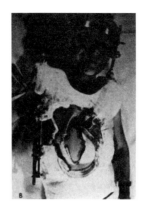 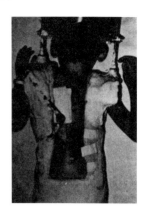

"HALO" ATTACHMENT TO THE SKULL

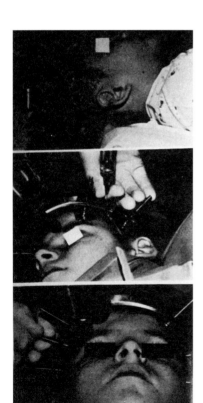

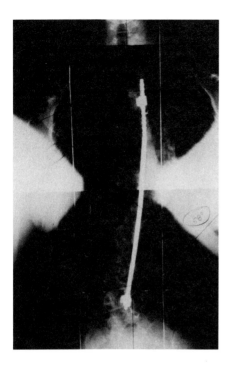 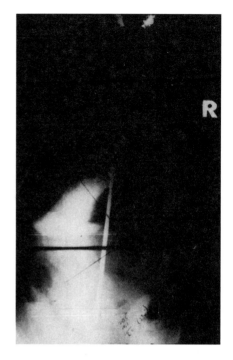

36 YEAR OLD FEMALE

44 YEAR OLD MALE

The above patient had the rod placement when she was twelve years old. She has been in constant pain, in the right shoulder and neck area for twenty years.

Patient had rod placement thirty years ago. The average reduction of the scoliosis is 30% with surgery. The surgeon did not reduce the scoliosis before fusing the spine.

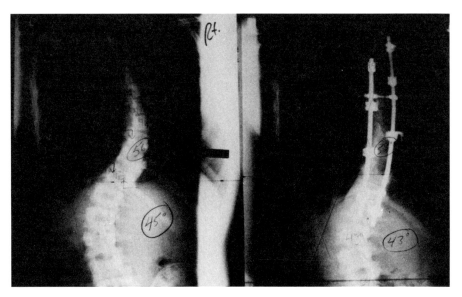

Double rod placement to reduce the scoliosis. In this case the rods were placed too high.

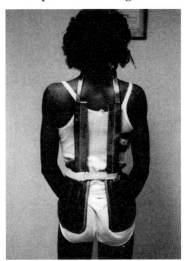

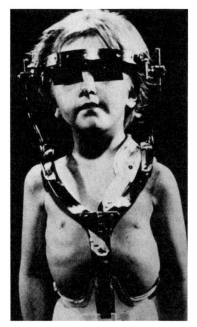

Patient wore brace for two years, twenty-three hours daily. The scoliosis increased. At right, body brace application on a two year old child.

I quote him only to make a point since I am sure there are many good doctors who would have recognized the damage these procedures cause. The problem still comes back to the point that the medical profession can not accept any new approach unless it has been completely tested by the profession itself. Because they are not trained in the area of spinal adjustment and biomechanics they will usually not test the procedure. This is the basic answer to the age old question "if your procedure is so good why doesn't the medical profession advocate it or at least recognize it?"

Medical schools are associated with universities. The university is made up of many schools such as law, humanities, dentistry, arts, etc. A college usually deals in only one subject, such as the chiropractic colleges. The colleges are generally private where we find the universities are state owned and funded. State universities receive federal and individual grants to conduct research and most drug companies carry on extensive research programs. In the last few years the chiropractic colleges have been able to receive federal money in the form of grants and are now working to produce the the research that will confirm what has been going on for a century. According to a recent publication of USA Today, congress has authorized money to be distributed to medical colleges on the East coast to help reduce the number of doctors being trained. Seems there is a surplus. Another case of your tax dollars at work.

With this in mind a medical doctor is presented with documentation, based on research conducted within their own profession, for the use in all of their treatment protocols. They are not encouraged to use any procedures that are outside the mainstream of medical research and therefore, when you receive a prescription it is based on research, and when you are put in a brace it is supposed to be based on research.

The Journal of the American Medical Association(4) in 1985, reported on the annual meeting of the American Academy of Orthopedic

Surgeons. They found that "despite widespread use of braces and casting there has been no substantial studies to prove that there were any clear results. All that has been certain in the area of treatment has now become uncertain." They previously felt that any time you had a curve over thirty-five degrees, you had to have surgery to prevent cardiopulmonary collapse. Their meeting produced a study that indicated you would have to have over 100 degrees to have cardiopulmonary collapse. After three days they came out of their meeting showing braces, casting and surgery do not produce expected results. Did it stop the procedure? I guess not, or I wouldn't be writing this book.

I have lectured, socialized and studied with members of the medical profession and have served as a non-medical staff member of a hospital and everyone I know has said they can not incorporate a treatment procedure that has not been instituted by their profession when it comes to treating scoliosis. Recently, I shared the podium with the chief of orthopedics of an Eastern Shriners hospital. We both presented case studies on scoliosis and discussed treatment parameters. He asked if I had conducted any blind studies on my scoliosis patients, and I told him it would be immoral for me to do so. A "blind study" would mean I would accept your child, and another one with a similar scoliosis, and set up similar treatment programs. Both patients would be charged for the "care" provided and results would be tabulated. The problem with this is that your child would not receive any treatment, even though it would look like it, and at the end of a period of time the results would be compared. To charge a patient for care they are not receiving is immoral. I could not tell you that your child was not receiving care because that would have an effect on the outcome. This type of research is conducted every day in hospital,s but I can not do it in my office.

The other problem with blind studies, in scoliosis, is there are no two scoliosis cases alike and therefore, the results can not be tabulated in a blind study. We measure the rotation of each vertebra and find that we may have similar curves, but the rotations are never the same. The marking of the rotations of the vertebra, pelvis, leg length and lateral deviations are what give us the direction in which the scoliosis is moving. Also how fast it is moving and how long has it been since it started. When the doctor suggests you have to wear a brace, ask him how long the curvature has been in existence and how fast it is moving? The only way to determine that information is by the actual measurement of the individual vertebra.

Another problem with braces is the treatment protocol indicates the brace is to be applied when the curve reaches twenty-three degrees. That would require a child with a twelve degree curve to wait for a year or more for the condition to become worse. If the brace is of any value, why wait until the curve reaches twenty-three degrees? Why not apply it at ten degrees to prevent further change? The reason they do not apply it at an early level is because the treatment protocol requires it to be used at a certain level of change. The doctor can not justify using it earlier since no "studies" have indicated it is a good idea. It seems to me the old adage of "an ounce of prevention is worth a pound of cure" still holds true. So, if the brace works at twenty-three degrees it should also work at ten degrees. The only problem is there have been no studies indicating success in the use of the brace, on all cases.

When we are dealing with children, withholding treatment is wrong. A case in point. In April 1996, I received a call from a mother in Oregon asking if there were any alternatives to surgery for scoliosis. Her twelve year old daughter was scheduled for spinal rod insertion in May and she wanted to be sure she was doing the right thing. We talked for over twenty minutes while I pointed out the use of the hanging x-ray, the use of heel lifts and the possible help conservative management might provide. We had doctors, who were board certified in Washington, and I wanted her to check with them. She cried because she was so confused since the doctors had told her that her daughter would be crippled if she did not get the surgery right away. When we finished talking, I could sense she was still concerned because these specialists had told her all that would happen if she did not have the surgery. In June, our office received a call from a man in Oregon asking if we accept memorial donations for our research. We said we did and asked for the name of the individual and found the name was of the daughter the mother had called about. She died following surgery at the age of twelve. The moral of the story is that it never hurts to try the conservative approach first.

This story is not meant to discourage, since we have hundreds of such stories in our files, I simply want to raise an awareness in the parents mind. As it has been said, "If you believe it is possible, no explanation is necessary. If you do not believe, no explanation is acceptable."

One brace brought into the health field recently has to do with the addition of air bladders and was developed by Arthur Copes. He has developed a brace that allows for the addition, or subtraction, of air in the bladders inside the brace so any changes brought about by treatment (chiropractic) might allow the spine to adapt. The one main problem with the rigid braces is any treatment applied may not have an effect since the brace could not adapt to the changes. The Copes brace is usually used in conjunction with chiropractic procedures, but we do suggest that any chiropractor dealing with treatment should be Board Certified. If they have only completed the Copes seminar, they are not board certified by the ISRC.

If a patient is aware of the types of braces available it is a good idea to ask the doctor why they are recommending a particular brace and how it would react to skin abrasions, skin rash, sleeping, etc.

Since the brace is to be working for a period of six to nine months, twenty-three hours a day, there should be ample time without the brace if the child is to have another x-ray. Too many times they remove the brace and take the x-ray. You must allow at least one week without the brace to receive a proper clinical finding to see if the brace was effective.

CHAPTER FIVE

TREATMENT PROCEDURES

I have eluded to the medical procedures which consist of "wait and see", "brace", and "surgery". The conservative management is applied when there is any indication a scoliosis is beginning. If we check a child and see there is a short leg, twisted pelvis, a "knock knee" or any other lower extremity problem, without evidence of a scoliosis, we immediately correct those problems since they are the starting points of a scoliosis. All conservative care is based on that premise.

If a child has a short leg or twisted pelvis we will usually see the child for a period of thirty to sixty days. We will start at three times the first week so we might receive a pattern of the weight distribution using bilateral scales. We have at our disposal a computerized bilateral scale that computes the amount of weight being distributed on the ball of the foot, heel, and each leg in an eight second period of time. This average is printed out so we may see the exact pattern the weight is following. In most cases of an acute case, the high weight will be on the high hip and in the chronic, the opposite will be true. We will also follow the four-step procedure which is "specific spinal adjustment, use of heel lifts or orthotics, exercise and restrictions." We will usually see the child about twice weekly for the next ten or more weeks applying any of the four parts of the four-step procedure. There may be little reason to work on the spine or maybe a series of exercises will help. If the child has a "knock knee" (genu valgus) we may work more on the muscles and incorporate orthotics. This will also be true if the child has any foot problems such as flat feet, pronation or supination. Medically, they usually do not check the feet and we feel this area is of prime importance since this is part of the foundation upon which the spine rests.

We class the scoliosis into six basic groups and have established a treatment protocol for all board certified doctors. These procedures have been in place for over sixty years and are modified as new techniques are developed.

Grade I
    The patient is accepted for a period of thirty to sixty days.
    Bilateral weight checks are made each visit.
    Application of heel lifts are made as the weight pattern is established.
    AP and lateral x-rays are taken and explained to the patient.
    The patient is restricted from physical education class to avoid trauma to the pelvis.
    Specific spinal adjustments are made to align the spinal segments.
    Exercises are added to their daily activities.
    If the curve is more than five degrees, x-rays are taken at the end of the thirty or sixty days to determine reduction.
    If the proper reduction is obtained, the patient is put on a monthly check-up schedule.

Grade II
    The patient is accepted on a sixty to ninety day schedule.
    They will be seen three times weekly for the first two weeks to reduce any symptoms they may have.
    The application of the weight check and the heel lifts or orthotics will be the same as Grade I. All other procedures will remain the same.
    There will be another x-ray taken at the end of the initial period and the lift will be in the shoe during the x-ray to measure the exact effect of the lift.
    This case may also require a hanging x-ray to determine the prognosis.
    The average treatment should take about fifteen minutes.

The patient may also be placed on a traction/distraction table to encourage flexibility and mobility.

When the x-rays are taken the second time a hanging film is also repeated.

If the reduction is as expected at evaluation time, then the case is reduced to once a week for three months and then twice weekly for three months before the next x-ray is taken.

Grade III

This case is accepted for ninety to one hundred-twenty days.

The patient is treated three times per week for three to four weeks, then reduced to twice weekly until evaluation.

This case also requires a hanging x-ray and the restrictions from contact sports.

The basic changes in treatment deal with length of time (total visits), amount of exercise and areas of spinal adjustment the doctor may apply.

There is the use of heel lifts and orthotics in each case.

Once the program is initiated the patient is doing 90% of the work necessary to reduce the curvature. The doctor controls the direction and the symptoms.

Grade IV

The procedure is the same as for Grade III accept there may be a larger heel lift placed in the shoe, as the treatment progresses.

We have indicated the following to be true in the application of these treatment procedures:

Scoliosis	Medical	Chiropractic
1-20 degrees	wait and see	80% reduction, 12 months
21-35 degrees	brace/casts	30-50% reduction, 18 months
35 + degrees	surgery	20-30% reduction, 24 months

These statistics have been compiled from forty-five years of case studies and indicate a general response. Each case is unique and must be handled accordingly. That is the advantage of the hanging x-ray, since it provides the doctor with the opportunity to see what reduction is possible. Each case is made up of assets and liabilities and it is up to the doctor to determine how the patient will respond, based on these assets and liabilities.

COST:

Doctor's fees vary throughout the United States so we can only provide you with a basic price which might be typical in the midwest.

90-120 days	Range
Patient will require an examination	$50-$100
Consultation	n/c
X-ray services (2 times)	$150-$200 ea.
Reports	$50-$100
Traction (20 times)	$15-$20 ea.
Spinal adjustment (20 times)	$20-$45 ea.

If we consider the higher number, a 90-120 day treatment period will cost around $1500.00. Based on the recent quoted price of $2500-$3500 for a brace, the price is not high when you consider the results that may be obtained. If a doctor sends films to us for evaluation and report, the fee usually is $150-$180.00. If the patient comes to the office for an evaluation and report, the fee is usually $250-$350.

EXPECTATIONS:

The doctor has the responsibility to inform the patient of possible results. We generally look for a 5-10% improvement in the first ninety days.

Medically, it is a success if a patient wears a brace for nine months and the scoliosis does not increase. If we can generate a 5-10% improvement in ninety days, this could imply a larger reduction in a year. Each case is accepted on a 90-120 day schedule until the first evaluation. If the response is as expected the patient schedule is reduced and another x-ray is taken in 90-120 days. If an expected response is seen at the next evaluation, the patient may be reduced to once every two weeks and evaluated in six months. Based on this procedure the patient will be x-rayed three times in one year. Many hospitals take full sets of films every three months which should not be accepted by the parents, since this is far too much radiation exposure. They do not use any breast protection and are only watching the development of the curvature, and if they are not applying treatment they should not be x-raying at that rate.

The Grade I and II cases will normally show a maximum decrease in the scoliosis within 12-18 months. If they are under age eighteen, they should be monitored annually until they are eighteen. If they are wearing heel lifts or orthotics they should be checked on the weight scale monthly.

Grade III-IV cases will normally take up to three years to reach maximum reduction in the scoliosis. After the first nine to twelve months, they may only be seen once a month, but it is important they are monitored.

Grade V and VI are simple cases that generally are under control in thirty days and do not have to be monitored.

Grade X requires the same schedule as Grades III-IV. The reason being that Grade X has a deformity at the fifth lumbar level and has to be handled as a Grade III or IV regardless of the number of curves the patient has. In this case we should monitor the case through the eighteenth birthday.

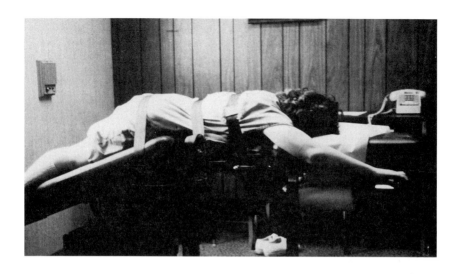

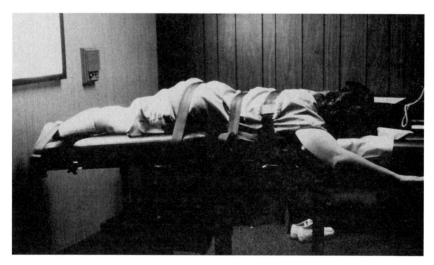

Traction/distraction table used for all Grade II, III and IV scoliosis cases. It decreases reduction time and provides flexibility and mobility.

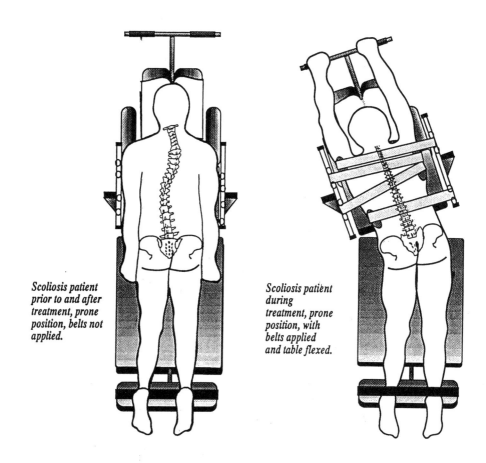

Conservative management of spinal scoliosis using the Leander traction distraction table.

CHAPTER SIX

AREAS OF TREATMENT

The term spinal adjustment has been beat up for many years, mainly by those who are not familiar with a spinal adjustment. Doctors, of various disciplines, have been moving joints for hundreds of years to relieve discomfort of one type or another. It was the osteopathic profession that initiated the spinal adjustment with their procedures after the civil war. The osteopath would manipulate all the joints of the body and use heat, water and ice to facilitate the effect. The chiropractic profession decided to incorporate the specific vertebral adjustment based on their philosophy of spinal interference with nerve transmission affecting the health of the body.

The actual application of the adjustment will vary with the doctor. There are seven ways to adjust a vertebra the same direction so each doctor will apply pressure based on their experience. If the doctor applies the pressure properly there should be no discomfort. Some doctors are very gentle and other doctors are rough. I have been in practice for forty-five years and have never seen a severe problem develop from an adjustment. There has been talk of people having a stroke from an adjustment of the neck. I have adjusted new born babies in the hospital and on house calls, and my oldest patient was one hundred and one years old and I have never had anything like that happen.

People who quote some off-the-wall statistic about chiropractors damaging the spine with adjusting, are wrong. USA Today reported in a recent issue that over 18,000 people die every year, while in the hospital, from wrong medications. Does that mean we will never go to a hospital? Anytime we deal with the human body there are things that can go wrong, but with chiropractic the chances are slim. Why else would our malpractice premium be so low in comparison with the other healing arts?

If the chiropractor has been recommended to you and they are board certified to work with scoliosis, you have nothing to worry about.

We recommend restrictions, while the patient is under treatment, to reduce the possibility of any trauma to the pelvis. This usually means no contact sports, horse back riding, bungee jumping, etc. We also restrict them from gym class since we have no control over the activities in which they may participate.

We recommend exercises which will always include the hanging exercise, some weight lifting, hiking and swimming.

There are no specific exercises that will work with all scoliosis cases, so we have the doctor tailor the exercise to the individual patient. When a younger patient sees the improvement in the hanging film, they are usually anxious to exercise for they can see what improvement can be accomplished.

We suggest <u>heel</u> <u>lifts</u> or <u>orthotics</u>. The use of heel lifts or supports deal with the laws of physics. If the pelvis, which is the foundation of the spine, is not level how can you return the spine to the mid-line? No matter how many braces you apply, no matter how much physical therapy you use, you will not reduce the scoliosis unless you correct the base upon which the spine rests. The use of heel lifts, to correct the pelvic imbalance, was started in the 1930's at Logan College of Chiropractic. Logan College initiated the first protocol for the correction of scoliosis cases with conservative means, that is without braces or surgery. The easy way to explain the use of lifts in scoliosis care is with the following example:

A sign post is along the side of the road. It is a large sign about six feet long. It is supported by two posts and a guy wire going from the top of each corner to the ground. The law of physics indicate the total weight be divided evenly down both leg supports. If someone brakes one of the leg supports the sign will lean to that side. The guy wire on the side of the broken post will become slack and the other one will be stretched to support the added pressure. If there was a round decoration on the top of the sign, in the center, it would be pulled to the low side, or the side with the broken post. Compare this, in your mind, with a scoliosis. One leg is short or the pelvis is unlevel (same as the sign without one support) and the spine (the round decoration) starts to rotate to the low side. Putting a brace on the spine would be the same as placing a block of wood against the round decoration to hold it from going further to the low side. Surgery, to place rods in the spine, would be similar to nailing the block of wood to the sign. Under conservative management the first thing that is done is to support the broken post, and that is done by placing a support under the post. In scoliosis it means placing a heel lift under the low side of the pelvis until it is level. With repair of the sign, once the sign is level new cement is placed on the new post, move the decoration back to the middle and the job is finished. In scoliosis, since we are dealing with a living structure, we have to increase the support in the shoe until the hip is slightly higher to allow the vertebra to rotate back to the mid-line. Once this has been accomplished, we only have to monitor the body growth.

Comparing the reduction of scoliosis with the repair of a broken sign can give you a realistic comparison to the types of treatment applied and the reason behind the application of the different types of care.

We suggest the use of <u>computerized scales</u>. The use of scales to measure the weight carried on each foot is necessary to determine when the proper lift has been placed in the shoe. We can actually vary the amount of weight carried on each foot by raising or lowering the amount of heel lift or support. The computerized scales give us a printout as to the amount of weight carried on each foot during an eight second period.

We suggest the exercise of <u>weight lifting</u>, particularly in teenage girls. We have found the proper application of bench pressing exercises can reduce a thoracic hump and in the early cases develop increased musculature to prevent the formation of a hump. Teenage girls have softer bones and do not have the muscle mass, so thoracic distortion is more readily seen. They also have a higher instance of sacral base deformity which will predispose to the development of a scoliosis since this indicates the foundation of the spine (sacrum) is uneven. The medical doctors are not aware of the importance of the sacral base and that is why most of the applications of care deal with the spine and not the foundation upon which it rests.

CHAPTER SEVEN
RESPONSE BY AGE

When teaching doctors about the conservative approach to scoliosis care I am always asked about the response at various ages. We teach assets and liabilities of scoliosis cases since each one is unique.

Example: Assume we are treating two patients, both female, approximately the same height and weight but of different ages. One is sixteen years old and the other one is forty. If all things are equal, physically, then the younger patient would respond faster. If the sixteen year old is a sky diver, because of possible trauma to the spine, then the older patient may respond faster. If the older patient has various osseous (boney) abnormalities, then the younger patient may respond faster. If the younger patient also does motorcycle motorcross, then we are back to the older patient. So all care revolves around the assets and liabilities in each case.

INFANTS
They respond very quickly since God usually does not make mistakes and the displacement of spinal segments, by the birth process, can be taken care of easily. I have treated thousands of babies over the years and an ounce of prevention is very true in the treatment of babies. Once the spinal segments are in alignment a scoliosis can not and does not develop.

ADOLESCENTS
As we said, our research has shown eighty-five percent are due to pelvic trauma in the formative years from five to ten. By measuring the rotation of the vertebra we can pinpoint the actual age of the scoliosis. We know the onset of puberty tends to increase the scoliosis rotations and when menses starts it to can cause the scoliosis to move faster. The majority of cases treated are with teenagers, so the response is generally within projected parameters.

YOUNG ADULTS
Their response is also based on the assets and liability theory, so their activities and postural habits determine the type of response we might expect.

ADULTS
The liabilities increase as we mature so the amount of response is reduced accordingly. We can still determine how much reduction can be expected by the use of the hanging x-ray. Some adults, with a curvature under thirty-five degrees, may still show a substantial reduction. Each case is an individual distortion and must be evaluated separately.

SENIORS
The older patients coming to the office for care are usually interested in symptom relief. There is little that can be done for a person over sixty years of age when it comes to reducing a scoliosis. The oldest patient we have worked with, that did show a reduction in their scoliosis, was a ninety-six year old woman(5). She had shown a reduction of fifty percent in her Vertebral Median Line Angle in a three month period of time. Since the medical profession feels a scoliosis has to be over ten degrees to be diagnosed, this patient was denied treatment for her back pain based on her age and the medical fact that nothing could be done for a minor(?) scoliosis. We feel any deviation from the mid-line is too much and based on that philosophy everything is done to reduce the laterality regardless of age. We have reduced scoliosis in patients of all ages and feel we may continue to do the same as long as we can determine the cause. There is no doubt a scoliosis will reduce less as we become older and that is generally due to boney changes such as arthritis and calcification. We will accept any patient asking for help.

SURGICAL CASES
We have always accepted cases who have had surgical intervention such as rod placement and fusion. Naturally we can not do any-

thing to reduce a scoliosis that has had rod placement, but we are able to relieve the pain that is associated with the surgery. We have had cases where the rods have broken, protruded through the skin, bent and become detached from the spine. All of these patients had been to their doctors and have been told nothing can be done except to possibly remove the rods. We do not recommend surgery under any circumstances since we have found all cases suffering from pain, caused by their scoliosis, can receive relief with conservative care. It is never a good idea to get a person to take pain pills for the rest of their life. We do not put a lot of pressure on the spine of a person that has had surgical rod placement. The areas of pain are usually located above and below the insertion point of the rods. The spine was designed by God to be flexible, and to allow for various positions while protecting the spinal cord. That is a general definition, but you can then understand what happens when you fuse over three quarters of the spine. The remaining areas have to do the rotating usually spread out over the full spine. This is why patients having the spinal surgery will eventually develop paraspinal pain that will be constant twenty-four hours a day. Many cases of this type, may have to be on pain tablets the rest of their life, but conservative measures can reduce the amount of medication needed. Once again, only deal with a chiropractor that has had postgraduate training in scoliosis.

CHAPTER EIGHT

CLINICAL RESEARCH

It would be of little value to the reader to have the expected research procedures and protocols explained. We have a variety of publications, in all the health disciplines, each one geared for a particular part of the professions.

We at the International Scoliosis Research Center have been submitting (case) studies to clinical journals that are distributed to the field doctors. The scientific journals are geared more for the scientific researcher than the field doctor. By submitting our studies to the field doctors, we have the opportunity to deal with the doctors who treat these cases every day rather than the scientist who does not conduct a field practice. In other words, does not treat scoliosis patients.

The following scoliosis studies have been published:
Scoliosis Related to Down Syndrome; Chiropractic Pediatrics (1994)
Scoliosis Reduced in Thirty Days; Chiropractic Economics, (1996)
The Efficacy of Chiropractic Treatment in Adult Scoliosis; Chiropractic Research (1994)
Chiropractic Treatment Procedure in a Case of Spasmodic Torticolis with Associated Scoliosis; Chiropractic Research (1990)
Vertebral Median Line Angle and Vertebral Pelvic Measurements Versus Cobb's Angle in Chiropractic Evaluation of Scoliosis; Chiropractic Research (1991)
Geriatric Scoliosis Response to Chiropractic Treatment Based on International Scoliosis Research Center Protocols; Chiropractic Research (1994)
Adolescent Spinal Scoliosis and It's Effect on Athletic Performance; Canadian Chiropractor (1998)

The next five pages deal with the advanced digitization of today's x-rays. This gives us volumes of information for treating scoliosis.

PROFILE

Name:
A/P Neut W/B [PV-C7] 07/11/1997
Age: 10   Female
Height: 5'5"   Weight: 81
Address:
FT WAYNE IN 46804
Phone: 219-432-7429
Treating Doctor: R. B. MAWHINEY, D. C.

COMMENTS

SUMMARY

Cobb's Angle	L3/T11=27.0°
	T9/T7=7.0°
Sacral Angle	5.0° L
Anisomelia	L-16
Pelvic Rotation	R-15
Stress Lines	T=2.7°
	L=9.7°

PROFILE

Name:
A/P Neut W/B [PV-C7] 07/12/1997
Age: 10   Female
Height: 5'5"   Weight: 81
Address:
FT WAYNE IN 46804
Phone: 219-432-7429
Treating Doctor: R. B. MAWHINEY, D. C.

COMMENTS

SUMMARY

Cobb's Angle	
Sacral Angle	1.6° L
Anisomelia	L-10
Pelvic Rotation	R-10
Stress Lines	T=6.4°
	L=2.2°

Spinalyzer Plus Copyright © 1992-1996   *January 06, 1998*

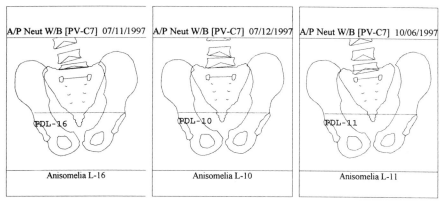

Strong leg syndrome is called anisomelia. It is constructed by drawing one line across the top of the femur heads while another line is drawn horizontally. The difference between the two lines is measured in millimeters. Some of the difference may be caused by pelvic and/or sacral misalignments and/or an anatomically short leg and should be correlated clinically. Anisomelia can cause subluxation(s), spinal stress, compensation patterns causing spinal dysfunction at higher levels, disc compression, and biomechanical malfunctions throughout the spine.

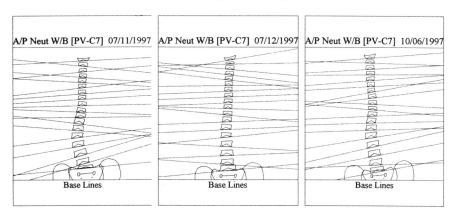

The A/P baselines are drawn through the inferior end plates of the vertebrae in the anterior to posterior x-ray views. In the normal spine, the baselines should be parallel. Convergence of the baseline is abnormal. Some possible causes are: Short leg syndrome (anisomelia), disc involvement, spinal fractures, muscle imbalance, subluxation, spinal curvature(s), subluxation(s), spinal degeneration, and congenital anomalies.

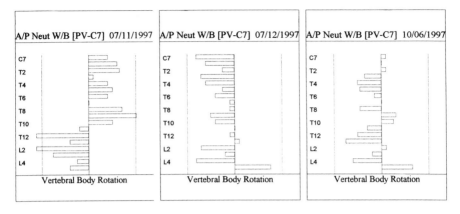

VERTEBRAL BODY ROTATION (VBR) is a measure of the rotation of the body of a vertebra from a true center line position when viewed posteriorly. Vertebral body rotation usually occurs to the convex side of a curve. Vertebral body rotation causes increased stress to the spinal system and is an accurate measure for determining abnormal compensation and failed spinal biomechanics. A relative reverse rotation causes excess shear forces on the disc and may compromise the integrity of the intervertebral foramen, as well as causing abnormal stress on the ligaments and osseous structure of the spine.

A/P Neut W/B [PV-C7] 07/11/1997	A/P Neut W/B [PV-C7] 07/12/1997	A/P Neut W/B [PV-C7] 10/06/1997
mm 20 10 0	mm 20 10 0	mm 20 10 0
T1 9.7	T1 6.3	T1 28.2
T2 9.1	T2 5.6	T2 27.4
T3 10.9	T3 3.6	T3 27.2
T4 11.9	T4 2.0	T4 27.7
T5 10.9	T5 2.8	T5 25.9
T6 12.2	T6 1.0	T6 23.4
T7 12.4	T7 1.3	T7 20.6
T8 10.7	T8 0.5	T8 20.6
T9 13.2	T9 1.3	T9 18.8
T10 14.5	T10 3.6	T10 17.8
T11 21.6	T11 2.8	T11 21.8
T12 26.9	T12 4.6	T12 23.9
Lateral Thoracic Deviation	Lateral Thoracic Deviation	Lateral Thoracic Deviation

The ossification centers of the thoracic spinous process are measured from a true vertical line representing the line of weightbearing. Any lateral deviation from this line indicates subluxation and failed spinal biomechanics or compensation for subluxation at higher or lower levels of the spine. Ligamentous instability and degenerative changes must also be considered as well as shearing forces on the spinal disc.

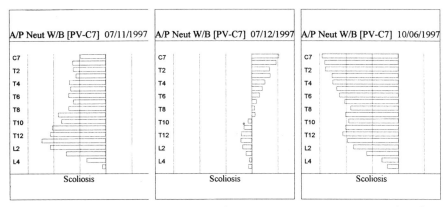

Scoliosis is an abnormal condition of the spine curvature as visualized in the AP dimension. Scoliosis causes stress on the ligmentous structure, interveterebral disc, the spinal musculature and canproduce severe deformity of the body, and in extreme cases, dysfunctin of internal organs such as the lungs and heart. The most commonmethodology for measuring this angle is Cobb's Method and the Riser Ferguson Method. From the chiropractic approach any lateral deviation from the midline with elements of vertebral rotation indicate a scoliosis with foraminal stenosis being present.

67

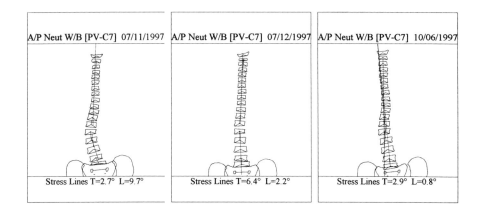

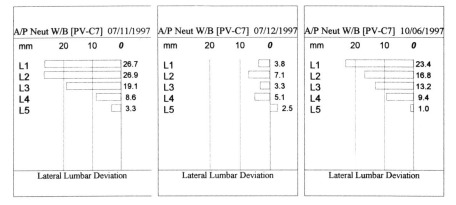

The ossification centers of the lumbar spinous processes are measured from a true vertical line representing the line of weightbearing. Any lateral deviation from this line indicates subluxation and failed spinal biomechanics or compensation for subluxation at higher or lower levels of the spine. Ligamentous instability and degenerative changes must also be considered as well as shearing forces on the spinal disc.

Actual cases of Spinal Scoliosis reduction based on treatment procedures by board certified chiropractors.

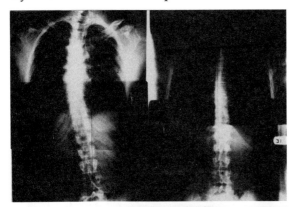

Antalgic scoliosis in adult male reduced in 30 days.

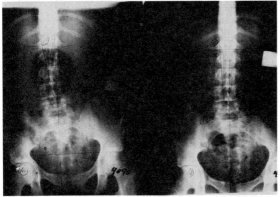

14 year old girl corrected in 60 days.

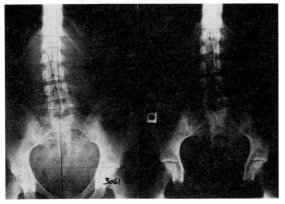

18 year old male reduction in 60 days.

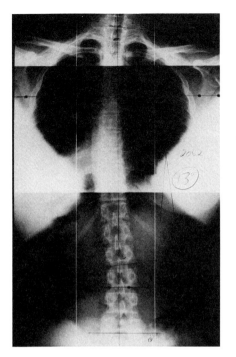 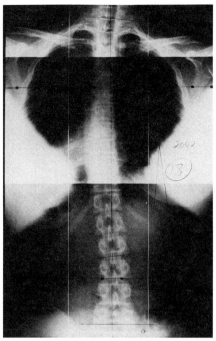

28 year old female 13° scoliosis — reduced to 3° in 60 days.

CHAPTER NINE

PATIENT QUESTIONS

The International Scoliosis Research Center receives over one hundred phone calls per month from all over the world. You are not alone in looking for answers to your questions about scoliosis. With the permission of the callers, we have recorded some of the conversations so you might see how your questions are the same as the callers.

TAPES:
The following conversations relate to phone calls received by the International Scoliosis Research Center. The calls deal with the type of questions people ask and what their concerns are in relation to their children and to themselves.

Connecticut: I have a fifteen year old child that is scheduled for surgery in sixty days and I am very concerned if I made the right decision to have the surgery done. I have called the American Chiropractic Association for information and they said they did not have any information on hand.

ISRC: You called the American Chiropractic Association and they did not have any information for you? That is unfortunate. I will have to call them and see what the problem is. To give you a little background, on the ISRC, I have been in private practice for forty-four years dealing in scoliosis. The ISRC was incorporated in 1992 to provide information to the lay public on scoliosis and to provide the doctors with instruction in the analysis and treatment of scoliosis. We do everything we can to inform the patients as to the options available to them in treatment of their condition. We provide evaluations on individual cases and set up treatment protocols for doctors to follow. We have never referred a patient for braces or surgery. We have reduced scoliosis and have published our findings in clinical journals primarily in the field of chiropractic.

The medical approach to the treatment of scoliosis has not changed in the forty some years I have been dealing with them. If the curve is less than twenty degrees, then they observe it. If it is over twenty degrees, but less than thirty-five degrees, they apply a brace. If it is over thirty-five degrees, then they suggest surgery. Our main concern is that it never should have reached any degree over ten without treatment.

Connecticut: Is there a genetic factor involved? Don't females develop scoliosis more than males?

ISRC: The genetic factor usually involves vertebra that have not completely formed at the time of birth and do not produce a firm foundation for the lowest freely movable vertebra, thereby encouraging rotation. Girls do develop scoliosis more than boys and there are a few academic theories as to why. The female pelvis is wider than the males and the placement of the lowest vertebra is slightly different and this seems to predispose to a curvature.

Connecticut: I would like you to send me a list of doctors in our area that I could contact and then get back to you for further advice.

ISRC: That will be fine, we will get it into the mail today.

California: I found this number on the internet and wondered if you do anything for post surgical patients?

ISRC: We are on the internet to offer help to patients and primarily to let them know there are other options to follow. We refer patients to doctors in their areas to provide consultation.

California: I am in constant pain, since my surgery, and I thought you might be able to help me receive some epidural shots?

ISRC: As you know by now this is a chiropractic organization and we do not refer individuals for shots. What I will do is give you the names of doctors in your area and you can call upon them to help you with the pain. You can contact us on our eight hundred number, but it would be easier for you to have someone closer.

California: You try to help people before they have surgery, correct?

ISRC: That is our main area of concern.

California: How many calls do you receive from people like myself who have had the surgery?

ISRC: I am sure when you read the e-mail comments you noticed almost all letters were from post surgical patients who developed pain at the end of the first year and have been in pain ever since. These are the callers we usually hear from and unfortunately, we are unable to offer them much help. We do provide some treatment, when possible, to relieve their pain.

California: That is interesting since I did not know that chiropractic could work with scoliosis.

ISRC: Our prime purpose, when working with scoliosis, is to bring the body back towards a proper balance. You have probably heard the term "idiopathic".

California: Yes, that is what is on my chart.

ISRC: This term means unknown cause.

California: Then that means my scoliosis has an unknown cause?

ISRC: That is correct and I ask "how are you going to treat a condition that you admit has an unknown cause"? The doctor applies a procedure and without knowing what caused it, is going to try and correct it.

California: That doesn't make any sense.

ISRC: We have found, over the last sixty years, that eighty-five percent of the cases are caused by trauma to the pelvis with posture determining progression. On this basis our approach to reduction deals with the pelvis and the posture which affected the spine.

California: Unfortunately it is too late for me to find these things out.

ISRC: I understand, but you sounded like a person that was interested.

California: I am now. Before I knew I had it I didn't know there was such a thing. I am forty-two now and it looks like I will be in pain for the rest of my life.

ISRC: Check with the doctors I have suggested and maybe they can help you. If the pain you have is above or below the rods in your spine, the pain is reducible. When the surgery is performed the surgeon will try to reduce the curve by thirty percent and when that is done it transfers the pressure points to above and below the points of attachment. The pain then develops in that spot.

California: I saw my x-ray and it looked like a vertebra was out of place. Do chiropractors put these back in place?

ISRC: That would depend on the extent of displacement and is best explained in person in front of the x-ray. In your case the sciatic nerve may be involved, which is the largest nerve in the body and if one leg is shorter, you have unequal weight on the legs and on the pelvis. We use bilateral computerized scales to measure the bilateral weight with each scoliosis case so we can determine when the pelvis is in balance.

California: You have helped me a lot and I will contact the doctors you suggested.

New Jersey: I am calling from New Jersey, and my son has a scoliosis. When I called information and asked for information on scoliosis they gave me your number. Can you tell me a little about your organization?

ISRC: I am Dr. R. B. Mawhiney. I am a chiropractor and one of the directors of the organization. I have been in practice for over forty years doing this work. (Note) Explanation about the history of the organization was given to the caller along with a description of what is done.

New Jersey: My son is six years old, has scoliosis and I wish to donate to some research.

ISRC: Our research is primarily in the area of case studies.

New Jersey: The curve was found during a health check and he had a thirty degree curve so the medical doctors said he had to be put into a brace immediately. So he is in the brace and nothing else is being done.

ISRC: This is where we feel the most can be done and I would like to refer you to a chiropractor, who is Board Certified in scoliosis, so your son might find a reduction in the curve. Bracing will not correct the curve, only try to slow the progress.

New Jersey: I asked the doctor about seeing a chiropractor and he said they don't know anything about scoliosis and it would not only be a waste of time but dangerous to take him. One question I have is this, "Are there any independent articles available for the lay person to read? I have gone to the library and all the books seem to deal with surgery or braces."

ISRC: It is true that there are not too many books that the lay person can read to get a better understanding of scoliosis. If you keep in mind that all actions have a cause and that the scoliosis is the bodies way of maintaining balance, it helps to understand why the curve increases. Many of the pamphlets you receive from various Scoliosis centers will describe the use of braces and talk about surgery, but none of them will be specific since there are no two scoliosis cases the same and therefore there is no universal treatment that would work with all cases.

New Jersey: Well, we are looking for a non-surgical procedure and it is difficult since we go to two doctors and one says wait and see what happens and the other doctor states that surgery was the only way to go. It is very difficult for us to know what to do.

ISRC: That is why the ISRC was put on line to help answer these questions.

We have published case studies on scoliosis. This has been done over the last forty plus years and in that time we have never had a scoliosis digress. If you understand physics, you will note that once the base of the spine is level there is no place for the vertebra to rotate so there will not be another scoliosis develop. These are available to the public through the ISRC.

New York: Doctor, I have been wearing a lift in my shoe that the chiropractor placed there and I wanted your opinion as to how long that lift will stay in my shoe.

ISRC: The lift is a tool placed in the shoe to enhance the adjustment of the spine, help to level the sacrum and to provide balance. The lift is generally slightly thinner than the amount of leg deficiency and is usually removed after the second or third x-ray to determine progress. If there is a measurable leg deficiency of more than one half inch, the lift may have to stay there for as long as one year. The x-ray is usually taken with the lift in the shoe so the actual effect of the lift can be measured.

New Hampshire: My daughter has a curvature of 46 degrees and I am trying to get more information on scoliosis. She wore a brace for about a year and even with the brace, there has been a dramatic increase in her curve. We took the brace off and I wonder if we should put it on again? I am trying to get other opinions, how about the Charleston brace?

ISRC: Each brace is designed to do the same job, but in a slightly different way. They are designed to prevent progression of the curve. Since God designed the spine to allow for graceful movement and full rotation, we have to remember that the brace only holds the spine, but does not reduce the rotation of the vertebra. By not removing the rotation of the vertebra, the brace becomes suspect in its use. When you remove the brace, no matter how long you wear it, the rotation of the vertebra will cause the curve to continue.

New Hampshire: Well, I need a doctor in Hawaii who could help. Do you have anyone there who is board certified?

ISRC: We do not have any board certified doctors there, but we do have sixteen doctors who have had some post graduate work in scoliosis. I will send you their names.

Kentucky: I have a seventeen year old son who was diagnosed with a slight scoliosis a couple of years ago. He began to do a lot of physical work and now his curvature is going wild. He has mitral valve problems, blood in his urine, refuses to drink water and only eats junk food. He is very weak and doesn't seem to have any strength.

ISRC: I think you will need someone close to your area that can work directly with your son and help him to understand the magnitude of his problem.

Kentucky: I am a nurse and we live in Kentucky, not near any practitioners of any kind, and I just need some help. If there are any doctors in this area of Kentucky, it would be helpful.

ISRC: The type of help you need is a little out of the field our doctors are trained for and also the patient has to cooperate since ninety percent of the reduction of any curve rests on the patients involvement. We can provide names to you in the area of Ohio and Pennsylvania, but you would still have to travel. It is unfortunate that the doctors in your state have not committed themselves to become board certified.

Kentucky: I know I can take him to Shriners Hospital, but I am terrified that they will do surgery on his back. Having been a surgical nurse there is no way they can convince me that is the way to treat his condition. Patients live with pain the rest of their lives and I know my son could not handle that type of pain.

ISRC: You may be able to work with exercises, and in his situation I would look for a certified message therapist who could do a lot for his musculature. The combination of the exercises and the massage may well restrict progression. See if you can get him to hang by his hands, on a daily basis. This will increase mobility and flexibility and also retard the progression.

Kentucky: I don't know how to thank you for the information you have given me and the time you have spent listening to my problems. I'm not use to doctors being willing to talk this long with someone in another state. Thank you so much.

Washington: Doctor, I have two girls that are twelve and fourteen years old and I wonder if they have a scoliosis. A friend gave me your number and said that you could give me some information since you do not believe in surgery.

ISRC: Please do not misunderstand, it is not a matter of belief in surgery, it is a matter of determining if results can be obtained without surgery.

Washington: It seems that this is such a common occurrence in girls that I began to worry about it as a mother. What do I look for?

ISRC: Scoliosis can be checked in the home, by a parent, much better than it can be checked in a school or other surroundings. First of all, do either of the girls wear a bra?

Washington: No, they haven't reached that stage yet.

ISRC: Have the girls stand with their backs to you, in their underwear, and look at their shoulder blades. If one is more prominent than the other you already have a curvature developed. Look at the slope of their shoulders. Is one higher than the other? Does their head tilt to one side? Are their underpants lower on one side? Look at the two dimples located at the waist level on the tailbone. If one is deeper than the other, there is a scoliosis. It is more typical in girls due to a variety of reasons.

Washington: That is interesting since my girls were checked out in school for scoliosis and they thought they might have the start of a scoliosis. I look the girls to our family physician and he said there was nothing to worry about. Now I'm going to look and for the first time I have a basis from which to look.

ISRC: This is what we want all parents to know so that they can check their children.

Washington: This is very interesting since we keep getting told by the medical doctors that there is no known cause for scoliosis. My mother was just diagnosed with ovarian cancer after she had been telling the family doctor, for over six months, that she could feel something growing in her and he said it was all in her mind. She has been told to exercise because of her arthritis. One doctor told her it was an inflamed stomach and gave her two pills to take twice a day. When they did a radical hysterectomy they found it was the size of two grapefruits and it had burst.

Wisconsin: I was wondering if a massage therapist might be of any help for my mother who is seventy years old and has a curvature of the spine.

ISRC: Yes, a certified massage therapist would be recommended in this situation. It should be a CMT or certified therapist.

Wisconsin: Do you schedule surgery through your office?

ISRC: No, this is a chiropractic organization dedicated to the treatment of scoliosis without the use of braces or surgery.

Wisconsin: This is a chiropractic organization?

ISRC: Yes. We have been working in the field of scoliosis for over sixty years. There are only two procedures for the treatment of scoliosis and they are chiropractic and medicine.

Wisconsin: Well I think I would like to try the surgery route for my child since the doctor said that if we don't have the rods put in her spine she may be crippled, never be able to have children and all of her children might be born with scoliosis.

ISRC: I do not agree with all the things the doctors told you, and if you want to stay in the medical field, you should get another opinion. I just want to say there is no way your daughter would have children with scoliosis simply because she had scoliosis.

Wisconsin: Well, that is what he told me and he must know because he is a medical doctor. Good-bye.

Iowa: I received your number from a friend and wondered if you could answer a question for me?

ISRC: That is what we are here for.

Iowa: My mother is eighty-eight years old and I rub her back at night. I noticed she has a large hump over one shoulder blade and it looks like a scoliosis to me. I took her to our family doctor and he gave her some pills, but she is still in a lot of pain. I have never been to a chiropractor, but I need help.

ISRC: As you are aware, as we age God designed the spine to become a little less flexible and therefore, there is little that we can do to make that spine flexible again. You might try a certified massage therapist who could give your mother some relief.

Iowa: I never thought of that approach.

ISRC: We deal with many people in that age bracket and our main purpose is to reduce pain and I am sure that is what you would like. I will give you the names of two doctors in your area and suggest you find one that will use a non-force technique.

Iowa: What about traction for my mother?

ISRC: We use what is known as flexion/distraction. It is to be used particularly in the younger group. I would not use this in your mother's case. If she does see a chiropractor, do not let them use traction. You may decide to use a combination of chiropractic and massage therapy. In a high percentage of scoliosis case we have what is known as pelvic unleveling. That would then be transferred into a short leg and when she is on her feet for a period of time, she will develop pain.

Iowa: I have mentioned these possibilities to her because she walks with a limp. We did not know where to go or what to do.

ISRC: We will x-ray the patient and then measure the leg length and place a heel lift in whichever shoe may need it. Medical doctors will not look in this area, so the patients end up with constant pain.

CHAPTER TEN

CERTIFIED DOCTORS

The following doctors are board certified in the field of scoliosis under the auspices of the International Scoliosis Research Center, Inc.

James Raker, 1305 Arkansas Blvd., Texarkana, AR 37757, 501-773-7246
Richard Matthews, 706 W. Quitman St., Hiber Springs, AR 72543, 501-362-8195
Steven Lukken, 13645 N. 32nd St., Phoenix, AZ 85032, 602-971-3050
Simon Yau, 625 W. College St., #206, Los Angeles, CA 90012, 213-617-8153
Chi Ho, 14291 Euclid St., D107, Garden Grove, CA 92643, 714-554-8899
Pamela Kirkwood, 1626 N. Main St., Salinas, CA 93906, 408-443-1222
Christia Nason, 943 El Camino Real, South San Francisco, CA 94080, 415-872-3138
Timothy Reilly, 1348 N. Center St., Stocton, CA 95202, 209-464-2225
Christin Bixon, 242 W. S. R. 434, Longwood, FL 32750, 407-834-2225
Michael Bagnell, 1544 Venera Ave., Coral Gables, FL 33146, 305-661-4303
Elliot Grusky, 11400 N. Kendall Dr., #100, Miami, FL 33176, 305-598-2005
Van Fotinopoulous, 2027 E. Edgewood Dr., Lakeland, FL 33803, 813-665-9597
Larry Johnson, 2717 Santa Barbara Blvd., Cape Coral, FL 33914, 813-574-5559
Maryella Gram, 2220 N. Tamiami Trail, Naples, FL 33940, 813-263-3369
Kenneth Carle, 5664 Bee Ridge Rd., Ste. 10, Sarasota, FL 34233-1500, 941-379-2737
Joseph Marshall, 411 Stephenson Ave., Savannah, GA 31416-0306, 404-981-4940
George Gott, 2308 N. Cole, Boise, ID 83704, 208-323-0836
Dennis Molloy, 201A Route 45, Vernon Hills, IL 60061, 706-376-7070
Sharon DeFrain, 107 W. Main St., Peotone, IL 60468, 708-258-9600
Robert Weckbach, 4805 Broadway, Quincy, IL 62301, 217-222-0399
Philip Gilbert, 517 54th Street, Huntingburg, IN 47542, 812-683-2215
Rebecca Jordan, 555 N. McLean, Wichita, KS 67203
Mikell Adams, 2032 W. 27th, Lawrence, KS 66046, 913-843-4114
Bradley Marten, 5000 S.W. 21st, Ste. 111, Topeka, KS 66604, 913-271-1113
Rosemari Wilson, 226 West Central, Ste. 112, El Dorado, KS 67042, 316-321-2273
Bruce Kempton, Box 214, Pratt, KS 67124
Terry Crow, 876 Third Street, Phillipsburg, KS 67661
Marisa L. Carey, Box A, Fruitland, MD 21826, 410-546-2225

Elizabet Stedman, 117 N. East Sreet, St. Louis, MI 48880, 517-681-2533
Natalie Dousette, 1311 W. 25th St., Minneapolis, MN 55405
Heidi Olson, 1311 West 25th Street, Minneapolis, MN 55405-2696, 612-374-3392
David Stussy, 1311 West 25th Street, Minneapolis, MN 55405-2696, 612-374-3392
David Tullos, 37101 55th North, Jackson, MS 39211, 601-981-2273
Holly Fink, 335 1/2 Second Street, Columbus, MS 39429, 601-736-5031
Kathryn Stanek, 403 Hwy. 43 South, Picayune, MS 39466, 601-799-2225
Brian Stanek, 403 Hwy. 43 South, Picayune, MS 39466, 601-799-2225
Dmitry Granovsky, 6 Garden Street, Seneca Falls, NY 13146
Gary Elsasser, 11906 "I" Street, Omaha, NE 68137, 402-333-0352
Scott Misek, 4852 South 133rd St., Omaha, NE 68137, 402-896-6131
Robert Flaherty, 1015 Main Street, Boonton, NJ 07005, 201-334-9019
Domenic Fontanarosa, 274 Lafayette Avenue, Hawthorne, NJ 07506, 201-423-9600
Glenn Strobel, 141 S. Blackhorse Pike, Blackwood, NJ 08012, 609-228-8888
George Bennett, 2193 Riverston Road, Cinnaminson, NJ 08077, 609-786-2222
Joseph Gitto, 6620 Ventnor Avenue, Ventnor, NJ 08406, 609-487-8787
Antina J. Balletto, 1700 White Horse, Ste. C-5, Hamilton Square, NJ 08690, 609-587-9500
Errol Toran, 825 Seventh Ave., New York, NY 10019
Jason Reznik, 1484 46th Street, Brooklyn, NY 11219
Edward Shnayder, 4000 Bedfore Avenue, Brooklyn, NY 11225
Alex Eingorn, 825 7th Avenue, New York, NY 10019, 212-956-5920
Mary DiDio, 326 Walt Whitman Road, Huntington Station, NY 11746, 516-673-1001
Anna Jenkins, 37 S. Hickory Street, Chillicothe, OH 45601, 614-775-0550
Byron Akita, 818 W. 6th, #5, The Dalles, OR 97058, 503-296-1900
Leonard, Caschera, 3811 Kutztown Rd., Laureldale, PA 19605
John K. Jones, 1 Woodland Rd., Wyomissing Hills, PA 19610, 610-478-1630
Paul Caton, 628 Darlington Rd., Beaver Falls, PA 15010, 412-847-2222
Randall, Kurtz, 116 N. St. Mary's Street, St. Mary's, PA 15857, 814-781-7117
Martin Gildea, 1010 Wesley Dr., #113, Mechanicsburg, PA 17055, 717-795-9737
Walter Zimmerman, 500 Roosevelt Ave., York, PA 17404, 717-854-4114
Benjamin Tanner, 871 Fruitville Park, Lititz, PA 17543, 717-627-1888
Mary Walters, 1174 Wyoming Avenue, Forty Fort, PA 18704, 717-854-4114
Marc Belitsky, 2633 West Chester Pike, Broomall, PA 19008, 610-353-2220
Joan Lee Rutenberg, 104 1/2 Forrest Ave., Narbeth, PA 19072, 610-664-4231

Yana Shenkman, 604 Washington Square South, Philadelphia, PA 19106, 215-925-8005
Zachary Weiser, 604 Washington Square South, Philadelphia, PA 91906, 215-925-8005
Dale Friar, Box 462, Isle of Palms, SC 29451, 803-971-0540
Gerald Liu, 811 Ta-Shun First Road, Kaohsiung, Ta R.O.C.
Mary Adkins, 1802 N.E. Loop, #410, San Antonio, TX 78217, 210-930-6937
William Ashworth, 112 Thompson Street, Ashland, VA 23005, 804-798-7575
Danene Saggau, 12911 Kent Kangley, Kent, WA 98031, 206-630-1575
Patricia Marsh, 10561 S.E. Carr Road, Renton, WA 98055, 206-271-6271
Susan Constantin, Box 1992, 2017 Main St., Ferndale, WA 98246, 206-384-4611
John Mishko, 7820 27th Street West, Tacoma, WA 98466, 206-564-2920
Stephen Chittenden, 10517 Gravelly Lake Dr., #27, Tacoma, WA 98499, 206-581-1533
Rodolfo Dabalos, 1442 W. Pioneer Way, Moses Lake, WA 98837, 509-766-9966
Michael Fisk, 1124 S. Pines Road, Spokane, WA 99206, 509-922-1909
Patrick Mawhiney, 615 Milwaukee Street, Delafield, WI 53018, 414-646-5657
Robert Mawhiney, 606 E. Wisconsin Ave., Oconomowoc, WI 53066, 414-567-1422
David Brouillette, 1624 Clarence Ct., West Bend, WI 53095, 414-333-4047
Gregory Gamache, 1624 Clarence Ct., West Bend, WI 53095, 414-334-4847
Timothy Baron, 104 E. Summit Avenue, Wales, WI 53183, 414-968-5212

CHAPTER ELEVEN

RESULTS OF CONSERVATIVE CHIROPRACTIC SCOLIOSIS CARE

<u>Before and After Films</u>

Each case A, B, C, show reduction of a scoliosis without a brace using procedure suggested by the International Scoliosis Research Center.

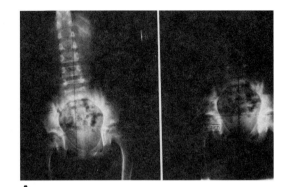

A

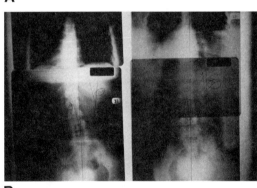

B

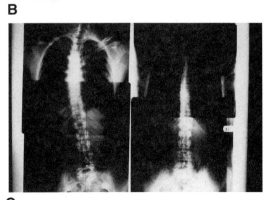

C

Young boy with Grade II scoliosis. Picture A.

Picture B is correction after 90 days without braces.

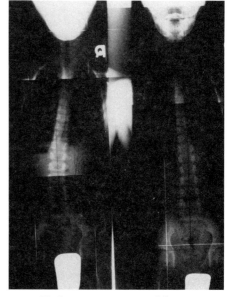

Before
A

After
B

Young woman with a Grade II scoliosis. Picture A.

Picture B is following 90 days of chiropractic care without braces.

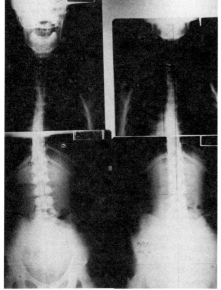

Before
A

After
B

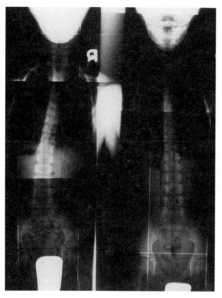

60 day correction
10 year old boy

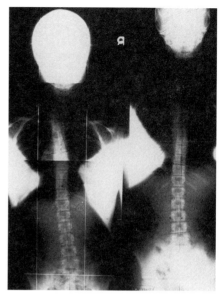

120 day correction
12 year old girl

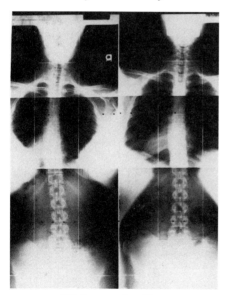

30 day reduction

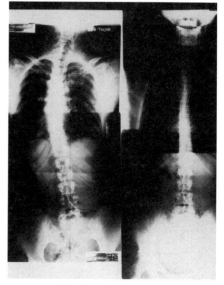

60 day reduction

(Left) Grade II right lumbar scoliosis in a twenty-six year old male.

(Right) Same patient in 30 days with conservative care.

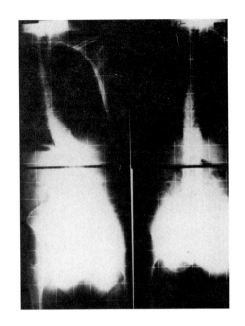

(Left) Grade I antalgic scoliosis in a seventeen year old male.

(Right) Same patient in 30 days.

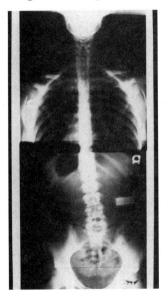 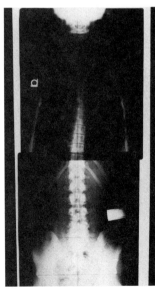

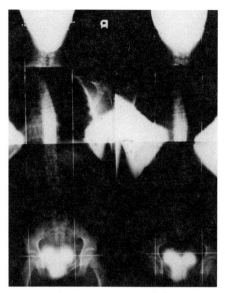

Antalgic scoliosis with Torti Pelvis. (This is a low back pelvic spasm type of scoliosis)

Before treatment   After treatment

SCOLIOSIS PROGRESSION

The picture on the left was after the first medical exam. They were told to "watch it".

The lower picture on the right indicates what happens without care.

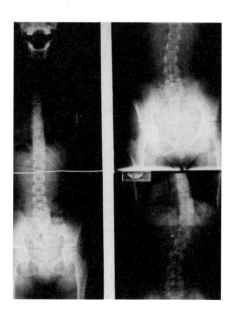

SCOLIOSIS BEFORE
(A.P. View)

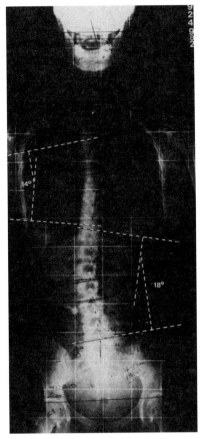

Female, age 26

Symptoms: The patient complained of neck pain and tightness, weakness in the legs and anxiety tension syndrome. She related that she had one "nervous breakdown".

Note: The next fifteen pages show correction of cases at the F. H. Barge Chiropractic office.

SCOLIOSIS AFTER
(A. P. View)

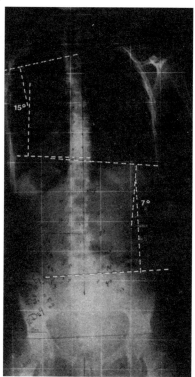

Use of Lifts: A 1/4 inch lift was placed first. Then a 3/8 inch lift, finally a 1/2 inch lift was used.

Comments: This x-ray shows a nice reduction in an adult scoliosis. A leg deficiency that created a sacral inferiority initiated this scoliosis. The 'pull up' L4 disc block compounded the inferiority, an indication of early righting reflex, upper cervical problems.

SCOLIOSIS BEFORE
(A. P. VIEW)

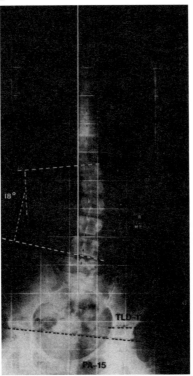

Symptoms: Female, age 25.

Symptoms: The patient related she had low backaches since age 17. She also complained of difficult menses. She stated that a medical physician had placed a 1/4 inch and a 3/8 inch heel lift in her shoe, but it bothered her ankle so much that she could not wear it. He placed in for her scoliosis.

SCOLIOSIS AFTER
(A. P. View)

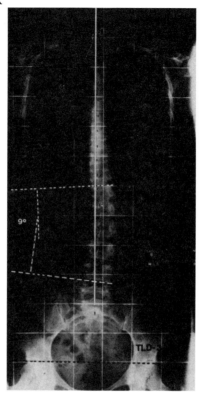

Time between x-rays, 8 months. A right heel lift was placed and then raised gradually until she was wearing a 3/4 inch lift on the right heel.

Comments: The leg deficiency, pelvic misalignment, and a 'pull up' disc block subluxation all combined to create this lumbar scoliosis. In regards to the use of lifts, lifts placed without spinal adjustment are often not well tolerated by the body.

SCOLIOSIS BEFORE
(A. P. View)

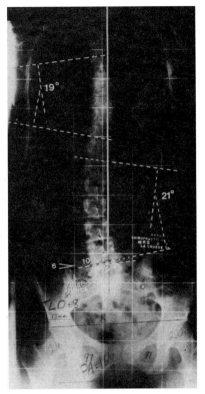

Female, age 23.

Symptoms: The patient related that since she had fallen down some stairs a month ago, she had pains in her right trapezius that radiated up into her neck. The accident evidently aggravated this scoliosis. Early chiropractic care could have completely prevented this scoliosis.

SCOLIOSIS AFTER
(A. P. View)

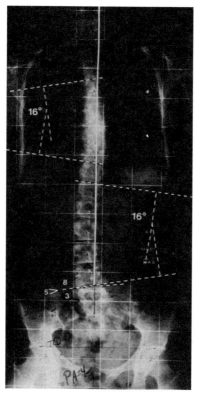

Use of Lifts: A left lift was placed gradually, until reaching a height of 3/8 inches.

Comments: Correction of the pelvic misalignment and reduction of the L4 disc block subluxation reduced this adult scoliosis considerably. Left untreated, this scoliosis certainly would have remained progressive throughout adult life.

SCOLIOSIS BEFORE
(A. P. View)

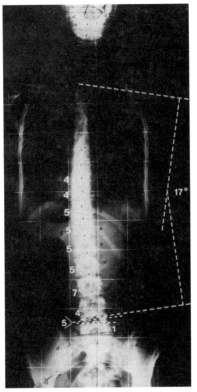

Female, age 20.

Symptoms: The patient complained of frequent low backaches, tonsillitis, and pain in the thoracic spine.

SCOLIOSIS AFTER
(A. P. View)

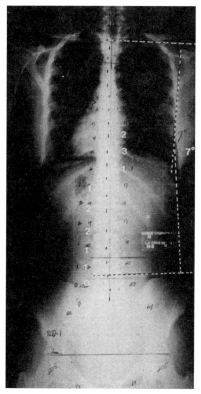

Use of Lifts: No lift was used in this case.

Comments: The patient related that she was in a car accident two years prior to chiropractic care. At the age of this patient, thoracic scoliosis is prevented by the rigidity of the thoracic spine and rib cage. The lumbar scoliosis however can be progressive. This typical disc block subluxation of L4, can later be involved in sciatic syndromes.

BEFORE AND AFTER
(A. P. View)

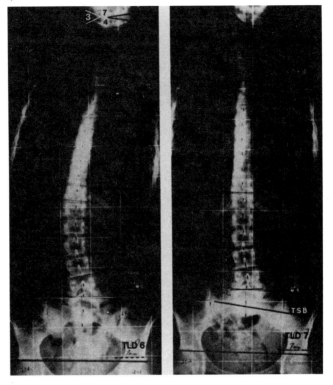

Female, age 15.

Use of Lifts: No lift was used in this case.

Symptoms: This case exhibits the acute scoliosis of torticollis. The patient related that before this attack she had frequent "stiff neck problems". Very frequently the symptoms of an impending scoliosis are felt by the patient in the upper spine as it attempts to balance for a lower back distortion.

SCOLIOSIS BEFORE
(A. P. View)

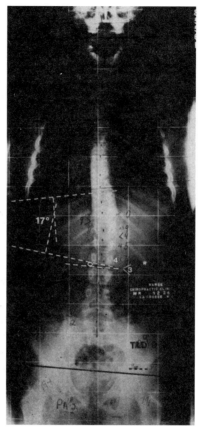

Male, age 12.

Symptoms: The patient complained that he could not bend over forward like he should be able to and that he had a low backache two months ago after a fall.

SCOLIOSIS AFTER
(A. P. View)

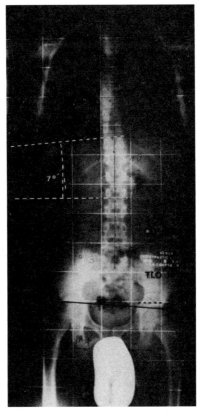

Number of Adjustments: 27.

Use of Lifts: A 3/16 inch right heel lift was used in this case.*

Comments: This, again, shows how an upper lumbar disc block subluxation initiates a thoraco lumbar scoliosis. Such upper lumbar subluxations are often traumatic, or are initiated by exercises such as sit-ups.

* Technician error, the lift was not in when the x-ray was taken.

SCOLIOSIS BEFORE
(A. P. View)

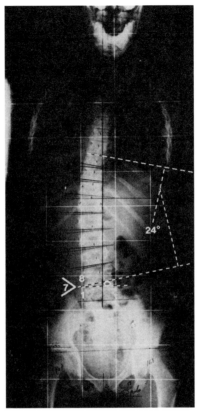

Female, age 9.

Symptoms: This patient was referred to us for scoliosis, she was symptom free.

SCOLIOSIS AFTER
(A. P. View)

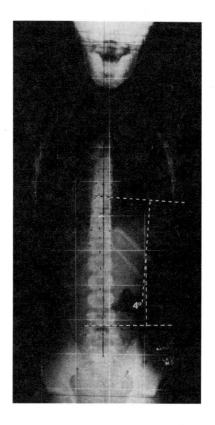

Use of Lifts: A 3/16 inch left shoe lift was used in this case.

Comments: The correction of the L4 disc block subluxation was of major importance in this scoliosis. As we have stated, scoliotic problems are easier to correct when a normal lordotic curve exits in the lumbar spine. The illustrations on the next two pages show the lateral and sacral base x-rays of this case.

SCOLIOSIS BEFORE
(A. P. View)

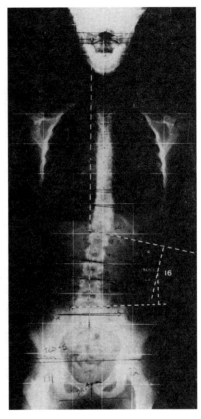

Female, age 9.

Symptoms: The patient complained of neck and shoulder pains since she was involved in a car accident seven months ago.

SCOLIOSIS AFTER
(A. P. View)

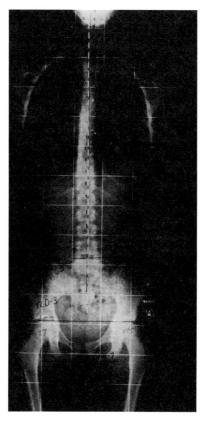

Use of Lifts: No lift was used in this case.

Comments: Both the righting reflex and a L3 disc block subluxation were involved in this problem. If chiropractic correction had not taken place, a classic thoraco lumbar scoliosis would have been the end result. The x-ray above indicates a remaining disc block problem, but not at the level at L4.

Graphic illustration of Hanging Films

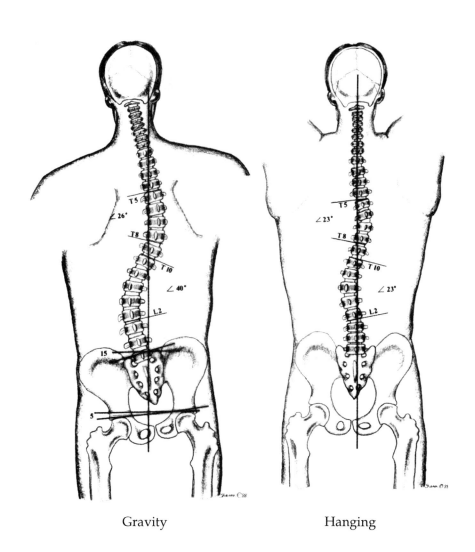

Gravity   Hanging

Graphic illustration of Hanging Films

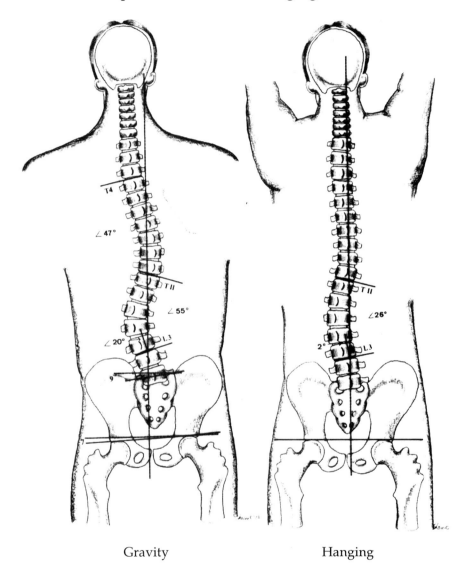

Gravity   Hanging

REFERENCES

1. Is Scoliosis Screening in Schools Missing the Mark? Mawhiney, R.B., D.C., Success Express, Fall 1985

2. Observations of Lateral Bending X-rays vs. Hanging X-rays in Scoliosis Evaluation. Mawhiney, R.B., D.C., Success Press, Fall 1986.

3. Points of Consideration in Marking and Interpreting Scoliosis Weight Bearing and Hanging X-rays. Mawhiney, R.B., D.C., The American Chiropractor, March 1987.

4. Scoliosis Management Now Subject to Numerous Questions. JAMA, December 9, 1985, Vol 264-#21.

5. Geriatric Scoliosis Response to Chiropractic Treatment, Based on International Scoliosis Research Center Protocols. Mawhiney, R.B., D.C., Chiro. Res. & Cl. Invest., Vol 9-#3-July 1994.